Chia

Also by Wayne Coates, PhD
Chia: Rediscovering a Forgotten Crop of the Aztecs

Also by Stephanie Pedersen
DK Natural Care Library
KISS Guide to Beauty

Chia

The Complete Guide to the
ULTIMATE SUPERFOOD

WAYNE COATES, PhD
with STEPHANIE PEDERSEN

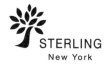

STERLING
New York

STERLING
New York

An Imprint of Sterling Publishing
387 Park Avenue South
New York, NY 10016

© 2012 by Wayne Coates, PhD
Interior design by Allison Meierding

ISBN 978-1-4027-9943-3 (paperback)
ISBN 978-1-4027-9944-0 (ebook)

Distributed in Canada by Sterling Publishing
c/o Canadian Manda Group, 165 Dufferin Street
Toronto, Ontario, Canada M6K 3H6
Distributed in the United Kingdom by GMC Distribution Services
Castle Place, 166 High Street, Lewes, East Sussex, England BN7 1XU
Distributed in Australia by Capricorn Link (Australia) Pty. Ltd.
P.O. Box 704, Windsor, NSW 2756, Australia

For information about custom editions, special sales, and premium and corporate purchases, please contact Sterling Special Sales at 800-805-5489 or specialsales@sterlingpublishing.com.

Manufactured in the United States of America

6 8 10 9 7

www.sterlingpublishing.com

PRODUCED BY
AUTHORSCAPE INC.

CONTENTS

One day in 1984, I left my desk to go for a run. It was noon, and not only did I want some exercise, I wanted to get myself out of the office. That was the beginning of my new, healthier way of life. As the years rolled on, I began running more often and at greater distances, until in 2000 I decided—for some unknown reason—to enter the Tucson Marathon. I ran that race and loved every minute of it. From that time on, some might say, my love of running got out of hand.

Which, I suppose, is where chia comes in.

Today, I regularly run 5Ks, 10Ks, half-marathons, marathons, ultra-marathons, and even 100-mile runs. Before the longer events I tuck film canisters filled with chia seed into my running belt. During the run itself, I dump about half the contents of a canister into my mouth, and then wash it down with a swig of water.

Chia is extremely digestible and soothing to the stomach (not to mention joints!). It helps with stomach issues, slows digestion, increases overall hydration, helps maintain electrolyte balance, and improves stamina during these extended runs. During these ultra-distance runs, some of which have taken me up to 32 hours to complete, you go through terrible mood swings, when you start wondering what you are doing. I found that chia helps lessen these gloomy feelings.

I'm not the only marathoner who's in love with chia: Many runners consume chia regularly, thanks to the success of the book *Born to Run*, by extreme runner Christopher McDougall. This national bestseller follows McDougall as he seeks out the world's most elite ultra-distance runners in order to learn their secrets. His quest takes him to Mexico's brutal, isolated Copper Canyon, home of the reclusive Tarahumara Indians. MacDougall learns their techniques and the secrets that allow them to run hundreds of miles without fatigue. Although I have not run with them, I have visited the area several times and run on their trails. The scenery is great, but the running is tough!

Having run both with chia and without, I now know why athletes love it so much. Chia gives you an amazing amount of energy and increases endurance to unbelievable levels. In fact, whenever I talk to athletes who use chia, they always comment on gaining more energy in the later stages of their runs. They also mention an overall increase in energy, especially later in the day—a time when many people grow fatigued and sluggish, and rely on caffeine and sugar for quick and unhealthy pick-me-ups.

Chia came into my own life by accident, really. I first came across this tiny seed in

1991 as an agricultural engineer. I was part of a team from The University of Arizona that visited South America in order to research alternative crops that might grow well in northwestern Argentina. Working directly with the growers, we planted a number of different seeds to determine which might perform the best. One of these was the ancient Aztec food, chia.

I'll admit that when my fellow researchers and I first saw the maturing seed, our initial reaction was, "What the heck is this stuff good for?" To find out, we began analyzing the seed to determine its various nutrient compounds, such as fiber. In the field, we saw that if it had rained, the seed would form a gel and stick together. This showed us that chia seed was great both as a hydrating compound and for retaining moisture.

Researching the nutrient profile of the plant, we discovered that chia seed contains an incredible amount of omega-3 fatty acids—4 grams per 2-tablespoon serving. In fact, chia has more omega-3 fatty acids and, in particular, alpha-linolenic fatty acid—the only essential omega-3 fatty acid—than any other known plant.

This was a hugely important discovery because medical research shows that omega-3 fatty acids reduce inflammation in the body and help lower the risk of chronic diseases such as heart disease, cancer, and arthritis.

Omega-3 fatty acids are important for everyday cognitive function (such as memory and performance), as well as creating stable moods and helping to regulate behaviors. Many Americans show symptoms of omega-3 fatty acid deficiency, which include fatigue, poor memory, dry skin, heart problems, mood swings or depression, and poor circulation.

We also discovered that chia boasts impressive amounts of antioxidants, including the phytonutrients quercetin, kaempferol, myricetin, chlorogenic acid, and caffeic acid. These antioxidants have significant value to human health, helping ward off everything from cancer to common viral illnesses. But what I found really exciting about these high levels of antioxidants is that they keep chia fresh and prevent rancidity.

Unlike highly perishable flax—which has an indigestible hard coating that keeps its nutrients fresh—chia's antioxidant profile allows it to remain shelf-stable for years. No hard shell means chia can be eaten and digested fully as-is. Because chia doesn't become rancid at room temperature, you can pulverize it as much as you like ahead of time, to use at your convenience. Also, chia doesn't have the slightly fishy taste that flax tends to develop shortly after grinding. These are three more reasons why my fellow researchers and I were so excited about chia.

But still the question remained, "What do we do with this seed?" Our first thought was skincare—the high omega-3 and antioxidant content make the oil from chia great for the skin. We also began feeding the seed to chickens and cows to create eggs and dairy products high in omega-3s. Beginning in the 1990s, producers began feeding animals flax, marine algae, and even fish derivatives to increase the omega-3 fatty acid content in eggs and dairy. Unfortunately, the enhanced products were left with an off-putting, fishy flavor that arose from the oxidation of the omega-3 fatty acids in the flax.

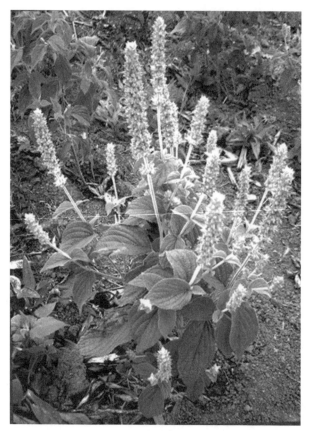

Our own research showed that chia did just what we wanted—increase the omega-3 content without altering the natural taste of eggs and milk. The amount of omega-3 fatty acids in the yolks of eggs laid by chia-fed hens increased by more than 1,600 percent, while the saturated fat content decreased by 30 percent. In a limited trial, in which chia was fed to milk cows, the milk had a 20 percent increase in omega-3 fatty acid content and a reduced saturated fatty acid content.

A member of the mint family, *Salvia hispanica* L. (aka "chia") is a pretty plant, with "heads" of multiple small delicate flowers sitting atop several stalks on a single plant. As the heads ripen, you can pluck off a few seeds and chew on them. The flavor of the seeds is pleasantly nutty, a bit malty, and very easy to like. However, it wasn't until I began an in-depth study of how the Aztecs used chia that I considered consuming it regularly myself.

Circa 2600 B.C., Aztecs living in what is now Mexico and Guatemala considered chia one of their most important crops. It was offered to the gods and used in rituals. Chia was also used as currency. The seeds were used in medicine, ground into flour, and consumed by warriors and elite athletes as a superior source of energy and endurance. In fact, it was said that Aztec ultra-athletes could survive days of grueling, intensely physical activities by consuming nothing more than a tablespoon of chia every few hours.

It is well documented that Aztecs were ingenious inventors of agricultural production systems. Because of their sophistication, it was clear to us as researchers that if the Aztecs thought chia was special, it must be. We read all the ancient Aztec codices, written approximately five centuries ago, that we could find in order to learn more about chia. A growing body of research made it clear that chia is a complete food, not just protein or omega-3s. Nor is chia "just" composed of antioxidants, vitamins, minerals, amino acids, and fiber. Chia has so many qualities and health benefits, in fact, that I am in awe. I don't want to use the word "miracle" to describe this little seed, because it would make chia sound trendy and hyped-up, but the truth is, I don't have a better word for it. Chia truly is a miracle food and, as some have said, it's "the world's healthiest whole food."

If there's one thing I have learned as a competitive ultra-distance runner it is this: You are only as effective as your health allows you to be. Chia keeps me healthy so that I can be at my best each day—no matter what kind of race I'm running, or what my exercise routine is. Chia helps me stay healthy for everyday tasks, too, whether I'm in my office writing scientific papers, traveling to oversee chia trials, in the lab doing research, or working on my chia website, **www.azchia.com.**

Two decades after my first encounter with chia, I am still researching the plant, the seed, and its many benefits. As time and money permits, I am currently looking into what else chia can do, studying its extracts, leaves, oils, flowers, and more.

My hope for chia is that more and more people will become familiar with it and give it a try. Chia really can help everyone—children and older adults, athletes and couch potatoes, people with acute or chronic health conditions, and even those who are currently healthy. In fact, I believe chia can improve the health of the world.

Keep reading and see for yourself!

Dr. Wayne Coates
Professor Emeritus, The University of Arizona

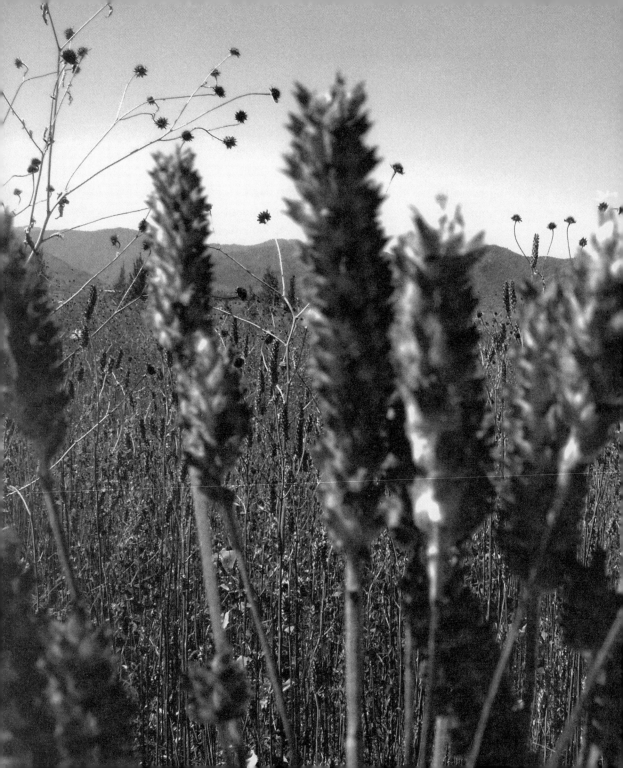

CHAPTER 1

THE MIRACLE SEED

Chia. This petite nutrient-packed powerhouse has been used by humans since at least 3500 B.C., when the Aztecs relied on it to keep their civilization healthy. Pronounced *chee-ah*, the small seed is currently making a comeback among athletes, nutritionists, whole-food enthusiasts, and raw foodists, as well as people who just want an easy way to lose weight, improve athletic endurance, increase energy, prevent a wide range of illnesses, fight disease, and improve the look of their hair, skin, and nails.

Chia truly is a superfood all-star. Wrapped in a tiny package the size of a poppy seed, chia is nonetheless loaded with antioxidants, vitamins, minerals, fiber, amino acids, protein, and the omega-3 fatty acid called alpha-linolenic acid. This small seed boasts so many benefits and addresses so many health conditions that many people feel it is one of the most beneficial functional foods around.

DETAILED ANALYSIS OF CHIA'S COMPOSITION OBTAINED FROM VARIOUS SOURCES

Primary Name	Sub Name	Specific Constituent	Average Value	Maximum Value	Minimum Value	Units
Calories			460	529	356	Cal/100g
	Calories from Fat		233	309	110	Cal/100g
Total Fat			30.86	34.3	21.4	g/100g
	Saturated Fat		3.47	3.91	2.48	g/100g
	Trans Fat		0.14	0.191	0.04	g/100g
	Polyunsaturated fat		23.97	26	16.2	g/100g
	Monounsaturated fat		2.36	2.76	1.71	g/100g
Omega Fatty Acids						
	Essential					
		Omega-3 (linolenic)	18.56	21.1	12.3	g/100g
		Omega-6 (linoleic)	5.93	7.15	3.88	g/100g
	Non-essential					
		Omega-9 (oleic)	2.12	2.71	1.41	g/100g
Cholesterol						
Total Carbohydrates			40.27	54	32	g/100g
Dietary Fiber (total)			34.43	41.2	30	g/100g
	Insoluble Fiber		31.39	35.9	28	g/100g
	Soluble Fiber		3.68	5.8	1.1	g/100g

Primary Name	Sub Name	Specific Constituent	Average Value	Maximum Value	Minimum Value	Units
Protein			22.23	24.4	19.7	g/100g
Vitamins						
	Vitamin A		53.86	80	30	IU/100g
	Vitamin C (ascorbic acid)		1.61	2.9	0.5	mg/100g
	Vitamin D					
	Vitamin E		0.74	0.74	0.74	IU
	Vitamin K					
	Thiamin (Vitamin B1)		0.62	0.79	0.21	mg/100g
	Riboflavin (Vitamin B2)		0.17	0.22	0.12	mg/100g
	Niacin		8.83	11.9	5.97	mg/100g
	Vitamin B6					
	Folate (folic acid)		48.53	51.4	43.1	mcg/100g
	Vitamin B12					
	Ferulic		64	158	40	mcg/g
	Biotin					
	Gallic					
	Pantothenic acid					
Minerals						
	Calcium		569.80	616	523	mg/100g
	Iron		7.72	9.78	6.27	mg/100g
	Phosphorus		770.30	880	675	mg/100g
	Iodine					
	Magnesium		334.50	369	321	mg/100g
	Zinc		5.68	6.48	4.46	mg/100g
	Selenium		55.15	92.5	17.8	mcg/100g
	Copper		1.66	1.88	1.44	mg/100g
	Manganese		3.28	4.32	2.46	mg/100g
	Chromium		9.07	16.4	1.74	mcg/100g
	Molybdenum					
	Chloride					
	Sodium		128	272	22	mcg/g
	Potassium		653	741	596	mg/100g
Amino Acids – Essential						
	Arginine (Essential for young, not adults)		2221	2750	1950	mg/100g
	Histidine		550	629	485	mg/100g
	Isoleucine		830	1100	700	mg/100g
	Leucine		1421	1700	1210	mg/100g
	Lysine		1005	1100	849	mg/100g

Primary Name	Sub Name	Specific Constituent	Average Value	Maximum Value	Minimum Value	units
	Methionine		609	1200	400	mg/100g
	Phenylalanine		1053	1350	900	mg/100g
	Threonine		735	894	647	mg/100g
	Tryptophan		452	1600	178	mg/100g
	Valine		985	1110	857	mg/100g
Amino Acids - Nonessential						
	Alanine		1082	1300	920	mg/100g
	Asparagine					
	Aspartic acid		1751	2150	1490	mg/100g
	Cysteine		422	500	370	mg/100g
	Glutamic acid (Glutamate)		3628	4370	3140	mg/100g
	Glutamine		3650	4000	3300	mg/100g
	Glycine		977	1120	830	mg/100g
	Proline		804	893	683	mg/100g
	Serine		1087	1280	928	mg/100g
	Tyrosine		584	880	25	mg/100g
Phytonutrients						
	Flavonoids (polyphenols)					
		Quercetin	35	60	20	mcg/g
		Kaempferol	35	70	20	mcg/g
		Myricetin	51	62	41	mcg/g
	Phenolic Acids					
		Ferulic	64	158	40	mcg/g
		Gallic				
		Caffeic	290	387	132	mcg/g
		p-Coumaric	75	102	40	mcg/g
		chlorogenic	603	1174	31	mcg/g
	Catechins (Flavan-3-ols)					
		Epigllocatechin	893	1850	90	mcg/g
	TOTALS		1599	2312	1106	mcg/g
	Other Organic Acids					
		Phytic	20	27	13	
ORAC						
	ORAC - Lipophillic		3	12	0	umol TE/g
	ORAC - Hydrophyllic		63	85	31	umol TE/g
	Total ORAC		66	89	33	umol TE/g

Table courtesy azchia.com.

FOOD OR SUPPLEMENT?

The Food and Drug Administration (FDA) classifies chia as a food that is safe for human consumption. Chia is anti-allergenic, meaning allergies to it are very rare. Also, chia doesn't disrupt human hormone levels, like other so-called "superfoods," such as soy and flax, which chia is often compared to (see "FAQs," page 150)

Indeed, one of the most common ways to benefit from chia is simply by eating it sprinkled onto salads and finished dishes, mixed into drinks and smoothies, stirred into yogurt and oatmeal, swirled into soups, and on and on. Wherever you might use chopped nuts, wheat bran, or flax, you can use chia instead. You can eat chia whole—the body utilizes the whole seed perfectly—milled or ground, or even soaked into a gel. You can opt for the more common black variety of chia (which has slightly higher antioxidant levels), rather than the white variety, which is less common.

Before going further into how chia can help you lose weight and get healthy, it may help to know more about the plant itself. Chia is a desert-growing member of the mint family, known as *Salvia hispanica* L. The seed is small, with a mild, nutty taste. Chia seed is hydrophilic, meaning it absorbs moisture (a good quality for a desert plant to have!). When a chia seed gets wet, its outer layer begins to swell into a slightly gelatinous covering. It's this quality (plus the fact that 38

THE HISTORY OF CHIA

There is evidence that chia seeds were first used as a food as early as 3500 B.C. Available to the Aztecs since 2600 BC, chia served as a cash crop in central Mexico between 1500 and 900 B.C. Chia seeds were eaten alone or mixed with other grains; consumed as a beverage when combined with water; ground into flour; included in medicines; pressed for oil; and used as a base for face and body paints. Aztec rulers received chia seeds as an annual tribute from conquered nations, and the seeds were offered to the gods during religious ceremonies.

According to records kept by the Aztecs and Spaniards, chia was traditionally cultivated in a region stretching from north-central Mexico to Guatemala. A second, smaller area of cultivation covered Nicaragua and southern Honduras.

The Salinan, Cahuilla, Sostanoan, Paiute, Maidu, and Kawaiisu indigenous peoples of the western United States used a different species of chia, called *Salvia columbariae*, for food and medicinal purposes.

percent of the seed is fiber) that allows chia to create a feeling of fullness (which, in turn, helps promote weight loss), while also controlling food cravings, balancing blood sugar levels, and soothing the digestive system.

As you keep reading, you'll find that chia's high omega-3 fatty acid levels have also been found to help the body lose weight and keep it off, as well as guard against a range of health conditions, including heart disease, stroke, cancer, inflammatory bowel disease, and other autoimmune diseases such as lupus and rheumatoid arthritis. Omega-3 fatty acids are molecules that the body does not produce itself. They are, however, essential in helping a large number of body systems to function efficiently.

This is where chia comes in. There are three main types of omega-3 fatty acids: Alpha-linolenic acid (ALA), eicosapentaenoic acid (EPA), and docosahexaenoic acid (DHA). Alpha-linolenic acid is the only fatty acid that is essential and is the type of omaga-3 fatty acid found in chia.

CHIA COLORS

Chia seed is black, dark gray, or, less commonly, white. If you notice brown seeds in your chia, you've got one of two things: grass and weed seeds mixed in (which can have a bitter, unpleasant taste), or immature seeds (which contain fewer nutrients than mature chia). To ensure that you get the most pure, highest quality chia available, choose reputable online sellers, such as www.azchia.com.

PROTEIN POWER

Chia is loaded with protein. Protein occurs in all living cells. Hair and nails are mostly made of protein. The human body uses protein to build and repair tissues, as well as to make enzymes, hormones, and other body chemicals. Protein is an important building block of bones, muscles, cartilage, skin, and blood. Our bodies need relatively large amounts of protein and must draw on it from our diet, since protein isn't stored in the body.

What is even more important is that chia not only contains protein (a generous 21 percent of chia is comprised of this macronutrient), it contains complete protein—an

CHIA PET TRIVIA

Did you ever wonder how the chia pet craze got started? So did we!

- Terracotta chia planters, in the shape of various animals and people, were long a tourist item in various central and southern Mexican cities.
- Chia Pet® is the registered trademark belonging to Joseph Enterprises, Inc., of San Francisco, the manufacturers and originators of the Chia Pet.
- Joseph Pedott was a marketing professional who, upon seeing the original "chia curios" in Mexico, decided to create an American version, which he eventually named Chia Pet.
- The name Chia Pet was first used on September 8, 1977.
- The first Chia Pet wasn't actually a companion animal, but a man. *Chia Guy* was created on September 8, 1977.
- The first nationally-marketed Chia Pet was the ram, marketed and distributed in 1982.

- Among the most popular Chia Pets are bunnies, frogs, hippos, kittens, pigs, puppies, and turtles.
- Chia Pets use the same type of chia seed that is edible and healthy.
- Joseph Enterprises also makes Chia Head®, many of which feature the busts of various American presidents.
- Approximately 500,000 Chia Pets are sold annually.
- Chia Pets are only sold in stores during the winter holidays.
- Chia Pets and Chia Heads are handmade pottery items. It takes an entire year to produce enough Pets and Heads for one holiday season.
- Chia pottery was originally made in Mexico. Today the pottery components are produced in China.
- Joseph Enterprises, Inc. also holds the patent for the Smart Clapper®, whose slogan is "Clap On! Clap Off!"

unusual thing for a plant food. This means your body can fully utilize chia's protein as-is.

The secret behind chia's protein power are its building blocks, amino acids. Do you remember playing with wooden building blocks when you were a kid? Plant protein is often missing one or more blocks, which means your body needs to find the missing piece in another foods in order to build a complete tower. Chia contains all eight essential amino acids the body needs to fully utilize its protein: Isoleucine, Leucine, Lysine, Methionine, Phenylalanine, Threonine, Tryptophan, and Valine.

CHIA AND MICRONUTRIENTS

Micronutrients are health-supporting elements also known as vitamins and minerals. (Macronutrients are nutrients such as carbohydrates, fats, and protein, which the body uses in large amounts.) Micronutrients orchestrate a whole range of body functions that support every single body system. Chia is full of vitamins and minerals, which help keep the body well-nourished and energetic, so that it runs at peak efficiency, without experiencing deficiency-caused cravings—which, in turn, can lead to poor food choices and overeating:

CHIA IS A NON-GMO FOOD

If a food is labeled as GMO it means that its genetic material has been altered through genetic engineering. It sounds shocking, but according to the National Agriculture Statistics Board annual report for 2010, 93 percent of the planted area of soybeans, 93 percent of cotton, 86 percent of corn, and 95 percent of sugar beets in the United States were genetically modified varieties. Furthermore, genetically modified food plants took up 135 million hectares of cropland throughout the world (in 2010). The Grocery Manufacturers of America estimated in 2003 that 75 percent of all processed foods in the U.S. contain a genetically modified ingredient. Chia is not one of these food ingredients. The seed, which grows well, ships well, and stores well, does not need to be altered to make it easier to grow or use.

Genetically modified foods are newcomers to the world's food supply. The first altered food was created in 1994 by a subsidiary of agribusiness giant Monsanto. A tomato was modified to create a fruit called Flavr Savr that ripened without softening (greatly reducing natural spoilage and bruising during shipping and storage). While the United States and Canada do not label genetically modified foods, other governments—such as those in the European Union, Australia, Japan, and Malaysia—require food sellers to do so.

- **Calcium** serves as the structural element in bone and teeth, and assists with cellular processes.
- **Iron** is present in all cells in the human body and is important for many functions, including carrying oxygen from the lungs to the body's wide-ranging tissues.
- **Magnesium** is essential to all living cells. Over 300 enzymes require the presence of magnesium to function.
- **Zinc** helps regulate many genetic activities. It also supports blood sugar balance and metabolic rate, and helps the immune system and nervous system (including the brain) function at optimal levels.
- **Selenium** is a potent antioxidant that helps prevent oxidative stress and inflammation, and boosts immune system function as well.
- **Copper** is a mineral that helps the body utilize iron. It maintains the health of bones, connective tissues, and skin, and also helps the thyroid gland function normally.

HARVESTING CHIA

Chia can be harvested mechanically or by hand. After the chia plant flowers, it is allowed to go to seed. The seed heads, on which the flowers formed, are then removed and struck to release the tiny seeds. The seeds are then packed into sacks or other storage containers for subsequent cleaning. No heat or chemicals are used in these processes.

- **Manganese** assists your body to utilize many key nutrients, including biotin, thiamin, and Vitamin C. It maintains normal blood sugar levels, protects cells from free radical damage, and supports bone health.
- **Vitamin A** is best known for supporting healthy vision, but it is also essential for keeping the immune system working efficiently, maintaining skin tissues, and protecting fertility.

Chia has become the staple of my everyday diet for overall health and well-being. I love that it's an all-natural food—and not a supplement pill. I don't miss a day of this tremendous source of omega-3's and fiber.

—RICK ROSEMOND,
submitted online to azchia.com

WHOLE FOOD GOODNESS

Chia seed is a whole food because it contains all its original components: the bran, germ, and endosperm. Research shows that eating whole foods can help reduce the likelihood of being overweight and can lower the risk of diet-related diseases such as diabetes and heart disease.

- **Vitamin C** is a potent antioxidant which helps protect cells from free radical damage, lowers cancer risk, improves iron absorption, and strengthens the immune system.
- **Vitamin E** is another nutrient that is a potent antioxidant. In fact, some researchers think it is the most powerful of the antioxidant vitamins. Vitamin E also allows body cells to communicate effectively and work efficiently.
- **Niacin (Vitamin B3)** helps lower the body's cholesterol levels, stabilizes blood sugar, helps the body process fats, and is thought to help protect the brain against age-related cognitive decline and Alzheimer's disease.
- **Folate (Folic acid/Vitamin B9)** supports red blood cell production, helps cell production, allows nerves to function properly, and supports brain health.

Chia has done so much for me. At the insistence of my nutritionist and health coach, I've been taking one or two spoonfuls of chia a day for four months now. My nails are harder and don't split like they used to. My hair is growing faster than ever. My skin is no longer dry and flaky. My digestion is more efficient and regular. My carpal tunnel symptoms have disappeared. And I just feel so energetic and great—like a younger, healthier, peppier version of myself.

—MAURA SULLIVAN, New York, NY

PHYTONUTRIENTS

Chia is famous for its phytonutrients, plant chemicals that contain protective, disease-preventing compounds. The phytonutrients found in chia include quercetin, kaempferol, myricetin, chlorogenic acid, and caffeic acid. Their role is to protect the plant from disease, injuries, insects, drought, excessive heat, ultraviolet rays, and poisons or pollutants in the air or soil. In other words, they form part of the plant's immune system. And what they do for plants, they can do for us.

Although phytochemicals are not yet classified as nutrients, researchers have identified these plant chemicals as important guardians of good health. They help prevent disease and have been shown to ward off at least four of the leading causes of modern death in Western countries: cancer, diabetes, cardiovascular disease, and hypertension.

THE BEAUTY SEED

The Aztecs pressed chia for its oil, which they used to heal and moisturize the skin, and also used it as a base for face and body paints.

CHIA IS GLUTEN-FREE!

Unlike cereal grains such as wheat, spelt, kamut, rye, and barley, chia contains no gluten. This makes it ideal for people who have celiac disease and gluten sensitivities. When chia is milled, the high-protein "flour" (see page 72) can be used in gluten-free baking. See pages 72–73 and 114–115 for gluten-free baking ideas.

AN ANTI-ALLERGENIC FOOD

Chia is remarkably anti-allergenic, meaning that most people (even those sensitive to several other foods) have no problem consuming it. A 2003 study performed at Southampton University and King's College London, found that chia has no allergy-associated properties. Furthermore, after studying all the available research and data to date, the researchers were unable to find any verifiable cases of patients with allergies to chia seed or any other plant seed that had a botanical relationship to chia (such as sage).

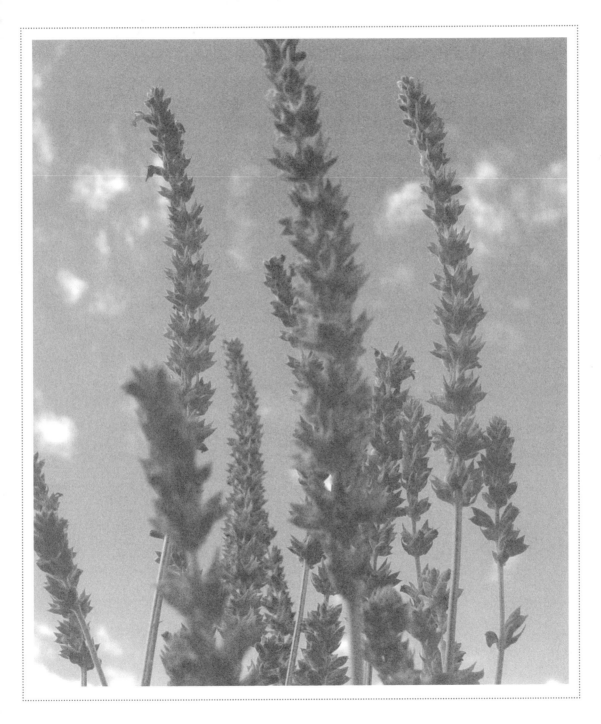

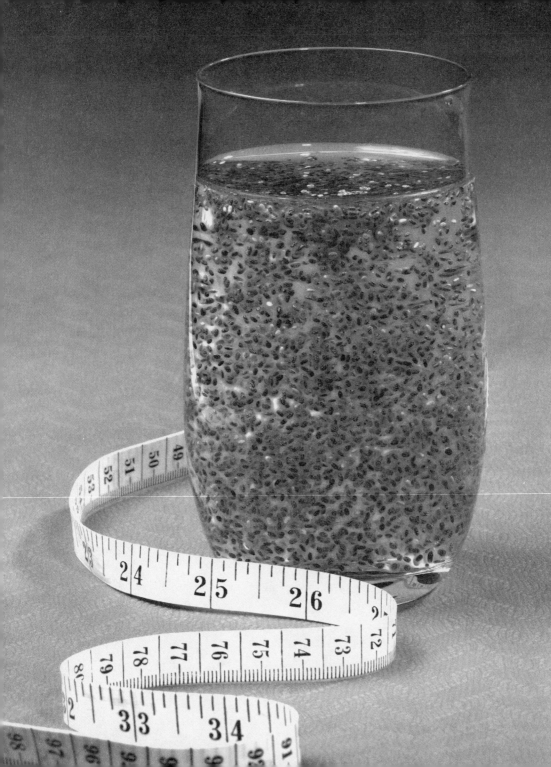

CHAPTER 2

HOW TO USE CHIA TO LOSE WEIGHT

Chia is good for so many health conditions and helps so many people that it seems strange to single out weight loss as, perhaps, the greatest benefit of using chia. But let's face it, we live in a time when there are more overweight people than ever before. According to the Centers for Disease Control (CDC), 33.8 percent of Americans were obese in 2010.

The CDC, as well as most medical organizations, uses body mass index (BMI), to determine obesity rates. People with a BMI of 25 or above are considered overweight. (To calculate your own BMI, look at *Finding Your BMI*, on page 24.)

According to a team of researchers at John Hopkins University, if people keep gaining weight at the current rate, by 2015, 75 percent of U.S. adults will be overweight. The researchers examined 20 published obesity studies, as well as national surveys of national weight and behavior to come up with these predictions.

This chapter will help you learn how to use chia to support your weight loss goals and gives you a recipe for success by adding chia to whatever you are already eating, if you are already on an established weight-loss program. You'll also find delicious menus that make it easy to stick with and benefit the most from your program.

WHY EXCESS WEIGHT IS SUCH A BIG DEAL

Non-pregnant human bodies are not meant to carry excess weight. The heavier a person is, the shorter his or her lifespan, and the greater their likelihood is of developing a weight-related illness, such as diabetes, hypertension, high cholesterol, stroke, cancer, sleep apnea, varicose veins, and others.

From a personal standpoint, being overweight means experiencing regular shortness of breath, having less endurance, and finding it hard to enjoy simple pleasures such as playing with your children or grandchildren. It means not fitting through a turnstile, struggling to find appropriate clothing to wear, getting stuck in a movie theater seat or behind the wheel of a car, and even paying extra for a seat on some airlines.

Then there is the cost to society. The more overweight people a country has, the higher its health costs rise due to weight-related illnesses. According to the CDC, medical costs associated with obesity are estimated at

FINDING YOUR BMI: THE LABOR-INTENSIVE METHOD

Finding your BMI takes a bit of effort, but knowing this important number is important to your health. Fair warning: Calculating your BMI requires using the metric system. If you have a metric scale and measuring tape, you can skip all the conversions explained below.

1. Convert your body weight from pounds to kilograms by dividing your weight in pounds by 2.2. So, if you weigh 150 pounds, that translates to approximately 68 kilograms. This is the first number you'll need in order to calculate your BMI.
2. Convert your height into inches and then meters. If you are 5'4" tall, that means you are 64 inches tall. Divide 64 by 39.37 to determine your height in meters. The answer for this example would be 1.6 meters.
3. Multiply your height in meters by itself. So, that would be 1.6 x 1.6 in our example, which equals 2.56. You are almost finished!
4. Divide your weight in kilograms (Step One) by the number you determined in Step Three. In our example of a 1.6 meter-tall person who weighs 68 kilograms, you would divide 68 by 2.56, which equals approximately 26.56. This number is your BMI.

FINDING YOUR BMI: THE EASY WAY

There are many websites that will calculate your BMI, most of which will work with a variety of measuring systems. Here are a few:

• www.cdc.gov/healthyweight/assessing/bmi/adult_bmi/english_bmi_calculator/bmi_calculator.html
• www. nhlbisupport.com/bmi/
• www.webmd.com/diet/calc-bmi-plus

$147 billion yearly. The medical cost borne by third-party payers for obese Americans was $1,429 higher than those of average-weight individuals.

So that's where chia comes in. Chia is an easy-to-take product that encourages you to eat less. It does this in a few different ways.

First, it fills you up. Literally. Chia swells up to 12 times its original mass in your stomach, making you feel full. It also lowers blood sugar levels, which can eliminate or reduce cravings for unhealthy foods.

Some research has also shown that regular chia consumption helps tackle "middle fat"—the fat that literally hangs around the middle of your body.

Lastly, chia increases physical endurance by "lubricating" joints and muscles and keeping the body steadily hydrated so it can stay in action longer without uncomfortable cramps. It supplies a slow, constant drip of energy so you can keep on jogging, walking, swimming, rowing, skating, or doing whatever else you do to get fit.

SPORTS DRINK OR CHIA?

In 2011, the Department of Kinesiology at the University of Alabama compared the effects of the carbohydrate-rich drink Gatorade with a chia-infused sports drink (half chia seed, half Gatorade) on a group of highly trained athletes. Both sports drinks contained the same amount of calories but a different nutritional composition. In the experiment, all of the participants took part in a 1-hour run on a treadmill followed by a 10-K time trial on a track. The primary finding was that there was no difference in performance between the athletes who consumed either drink. In other words, the "chia sports drink" was just as effective as the straight Gatorade. There's a good chance that agua fresca (see page 65) would perform just as well, allowing athletes to reduce their intake of sugar and chemical ingredients even further, while increasing fiber, protein, antioxidants, and omega-3 fatty acids.

THE CHIA PLAN HOW-TO'S

These are the golden rules for using chia to support your weight loss goals:

- **Ditch the junk.** If you are eating potato chips and chocolate chip cookies, chia may not help you lose weight. Choose fruit, vegetables, whole grains, and lean proteins instead.
- **Drink 8 to 12 glasses of water a day.** Chia is hydrophilic, meaning it absorbs water. Give it the water it needs to do its job.
- **Watch portion sizes.** One 3-ounce serving of animal protein (fish, poultry, or red meat) is the size of a deck of cards. Most people get much, much, more than this. A serving of fruit is generally one medium-sized piece.
- **Include plant protein in your diet.** Good sources include beans, dried peas, quinoa, amaranth, nuts (including nut butters), and chia.
- **Cut down or cut out alcohol.** Alcohol is a high-calorie beverage with a number of weight loss drawbacks that have been shown to raise blood sugar levels, leading to cravings. Alcohol can lessen judgment, which can cause you to eat more than you normally would. In fact, one study found that people typically consumed 20 percent more calories at a meal when they had drunk alcohol beforehand. There was a total caloric increase of 33 percent when the calories from the alcohol were added. Along

CHIA CURBS CRAVINGS

The January 2010 issue of the *European Journal of Clinical Nutrition* features a study on 11 healthy-weight men and women. For 12 weeks, test subjects consumed 0, 7, 15, or 24 grams of chia. Blood samples and appetite ratings were taken several times within two hours after consuming chia. The findings? Sugar levels were decreased in everyone who consumed chia, regardless of the dose. Appetite ratings were also significantly decreased, even at 120 minutes after consuming chia. Intriguingly, many people who eat chia regularly report that it "takes the edge" off their hunger, allowing them to be satiated with less food.

with the increase in weight you can have an increased risk to your health because of *where* you gain the weight. A study of over 3,000 people showed that consuming elevated amounts of alcohol is associated with abdominal obesity in men. Many people jokingly term this weight gain a "beer belly."

- **Limit caffeine.** Drinking the equivalent of two cups of coffee daily can set you up for high blood sugar levels, which in turn can lead to strong cravings for sugary, starchy (read: fattening) foods. How? Caffeine tells the hormones glucogen and adrenaline to release sugar stored in the liver. The result? High blood glucose.
- **Increase vegetables.** Your body deserves the rich bounty of vitamins, minerals, fiber, and phytonutrients these wonderful foods offer.
- **Cut out diet sodas.** A study by the American Diabetes Association (ADA) has found that individuals who drink diet sodas are heavier, on average, than individuals who don't. The ADA analyzed measures of height, weight, and waist circumference compared to diet soda consumption over a period of nine and a half years and found that adults who drank larger quantities of diet soda per day gained more weight and added more to their waistline than adults who don't drink diet sodas. The study shows that while diet sodas may be free of calories, they do not prevent you from gaining weight. Diet soda also contributes to diabetes, heart disease, cancer, and other chronic

conditions. A study by the American Stroke Association discovered that individuals who had one diet soda every day had a 61 percent higher risk of "cardiovascular events," such as stroke and heart attack, than those who never drink diet sodas.

- **Cut out regular sodas.** One 12-ounce can of soda has anywhere from 140 to 165 calories, plus loads of artificial ingredients your body doesn't need. It's better to drink water—with or without chia seed mixed in.

- **Ban hydrogenated fats,** also known as trans fats, from your diet. These are industrially-made fats that are used to increase shelf life in convenience and snack foods. Studies have found that trans fats harden arteries, raise cholesterol levels, and increase the risk of heart disease.

- **Go easy on fruit juice.** It has a lot of calories and is pure fruit sugar.

- **Get moving!** Go to Chapter Four (see page 49) and choose an exercise program. Plan on exercising regularly to lose weight and tone your muscles.

HOW OUR DIETS HAVE CHANGED

Back before electricity, plumbing, and perhaps even before the wheel, humans ate much differently than they do today. One of the most dramatic changes to the human diet has been the ratio between omega-6 and omega-3 essential fatty acids (EFA). Our bodies require both of these EFAs. However, our diet today consists of much more omega-6 fatty acids, which are found in grain-fed poultry and meat, and industrially-produced cooking oils, such as safflower and canola oils, as well as corn and soy products, then it did during our evolutionary period.

Historically, during the hunter and gatherer era, this balance was 1:1 or even 1:2 in favor of omega-3 fatty acids, the fatty acids that come from plant food and animals that eat wild plant food.

Today, this balance has shifted to 10:1 or even 20:1! What this means is that we consume 10 or 20 times more omega-6 fatty acids than omega-3s.

Why is this a problem? Research has shown that too high a ratio of omega-6 to omega-3 fatty acids can cause heart disease, along with a host of other illnesses. Most likely, this is because omega-6 fatty acids have inflammatory properties, while omega-3s are anti-inflammatory. With the high dose of omega-6 fatty acids that we consume, it is likely that most of us experience some sort of inflammation, the root of many health issues.

SUPPORTING POPULAR DIET PROGRAMS

If you are already on any established weight loss program—such as Weight Watchers, The Zone, The Blood Type Diet, Atkins, or Jenny Craig—chia can be just what you need to ensure success. Simply adding chia to what you are already eating can help fill you up, create a feeling of satiety—so you won't eat more than you need—and help regulate blood sugar levels, so you won't be waylaid by cravings for sugary or starchy foods. Here is a recipe for success:

PHASE ONE:

In this phase, you are easing into chia and getting your body acclimated to the extra dose of fiber chia provides. For every step listed below in Phase One, Two, and Three, you can either sprinkle chia onto your food or stir it into your food. If preferred, you could

BRAIN FOOD

Chia is rich in alpha-linolenic acid, the only essential omega-3 fatty acid. Also known as EFAs, these nutrients are known to make cell membranes more flexible and efficient, making nutrients more readily available and nerve transmission more efficient. This helps to improve mood, memory, and brain function.

also mix it into a small glass of water or juice and drink it. Plan on staying in this phase for two weeks before moving to Phase Two:

• **Breakfast:** ½ tablespoon whole chia seed or milled chia with breakfast.
• **Lunch:** ½ tablespoon whole chia seed or milled chia with lunch.
• **Dinner:** ½ tablespoon whole chia seed or milled chia with dinner.

My experience with chia has been very positive. About a year ago I started, sprinkling a large spoonful every day on my dinner salad. What I discovered is that I no longer had the desire to eat my 9:00 p.m. bowl of ice cream. My stomach was pleasantly full and I just didn't crave it like I once did. After a few months, I began adding a spoonful into my breakfast smoothie and I found that I no longer wanted my 10:30 a.m. granola bar. Just a month ago, I added a third spoonful, this one at lunch. What I've noticed is instead of craving chips or a Snickers bar at 3:00 p.m., I now am happy with a tomato or vegetable juice. These aren't huge changes, but they've added up to a 17-pound weight loss without changing what I like to eat for breakfast, lunch, and dinner.

—SARA CARAVILLE, Seattle, WA

PHASE TWO:

In this phase, your body is comfortable with chia so it's a great time to add more. You'll see an increase in benefits as well as experiencing greater satiety at mealtime. Plan on being in Phase Two for one month before moving onto Phase Three.

• **Breakfast:** ½ tablespoon whole chia seed or milled chia with breakfast.

• **Midmorning snack:** ½ tablespoon whole chia seed or milled chia with snack.

• **Lunch:** ½ tablespoon whole chia seed or milled chia with lunch.

• **Afternoon snack:** ½ tablespoon whole chia seed or milled chia with snack.

• **Dinner:** ½ tablespoon whole chia seed or milled chia with dinner.

SLIMMER AND HEALTHIER WITH CHIA

The place was the Twenty-Fourth International Symposium on Diabetes and Nutrition of the European Association for the Study of Diabetes, held in Salerno, Italy, in June 2004. What had everyone so excited? The University of Antwerp in Belgium presented research findings for its "chia study." For a full month, researchers gave healthy individuals 45 grams of chia (a bit under 4 tablespoons) every single day. The result? A reduction in blood pressure and triglycerides, plus smaller waist circumference and less abdominal fat.

PHASE THREE:

In this phase, you reach the 45 daily grams of chia that researchers have found best supports weight loss and maintenance. You'll see an increase in health benefits as well as experiencing greater satiety at mealtime. Plan on staying in Phase Three until you reach your goal weight.

• **Breakfast:** 1 tablespoon whole chia seed or milled chia with breakfast.

• **Midmorning snack:** ½ tablespoon whole chia seed or milled chia with snack.

• **Lunch:** 1 tablespoon whole chia seed or milled chia with lunch.

• **Afternoon snack:** ½ tablespoon whole chia seed or milled chia with snack.

• **Dinner:** 1 tablespoon whole chia seed or milled chia with dinner.

I've been eating chia seed every day for about a year and a half. Nine months ago, I had my cholesterol checked and it had gone down from 204 the year before to 178. I had been trying to get my cholesterol down below 200 for three years by eating well, to no avail. I bet it goes down even further when I get my blood work done again in January. I also bake with it and use it on my long-distance runs as energy. It is a wonderful endurance food for athletes.

—RENEE STEVENS,
posted online at azchia.com

HIGH FIBER FOODS

Fill up on fiber and you're less likely to fill up on fatty, sugary foods that compromise your weight loss efforts. Here are some favorites:

- **Chia:** One tablespoon has 5000 mg or 5 grams of total fiber
- **Avocado:** One medium avocado contains 11 grams of fiber.
- **Artichoke:** A medium artichoke boasts 10 grams of fiber.
- **Raspberries:** A cup of these red berries contains 8 grams of fiber.
- **Blackberries:** A cup of these "bramble fruits" contains 8 grams of fiber.
- **Lentils:** These legumes are not only rich in protein, a half-cup serving contains 8 grams of fiber.
- **Black beans:** An all-around favorite, black beans contain 7 grams of fiber per half-cup.
- **Broccoli:** A cup of this brassica-family favorite boasts 6 grams of fiber.
- **Pear:** One medium pear has 4.5 grams of fiber.
- **Apple:** Choose your favorite variety! One medium piece of this fruit provides 4 grams of fiber.
- **Almonds:** A ¼ cup serving offers up 4.25 grams of fiber.
- **Sesame seeds:** One ounce offers 4 grams of fiber.
- **Coconut flakes:** Choose 1 ounce of unsweetened coconut and you get 5 grams of fiber.

OPTIONAL ONE-WEEK MENUS You do not need formal recipes to enjoy chia, nor do you need a menu plan to use chia as a weight loss support. All you need to do is read *The Chia Plan How-To's* on page 25, since the chia weight-loss "program" simply consists of choosing healthy foods, adding chia (as described in *Supporting Popular Diet Programs* on page 28), and exercising regularly.

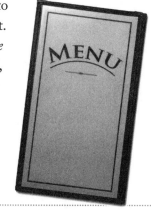

If you enjoy following recipes, however, and find that they make it easier and more enjoyable to achieve your weight loss and health goals, take a look at Chapter 5: "Cooking, Eating, and Healing with Chia" on page 65 for some delicious examples.

You'll notice there are three phases. This is to get your body used to the amount of chia you'll be taking in.

PHASE ONE MENUS:

In this phase, you are easing into chia and getting your body acclimated to the extra dose of fiber chia provides. Plan on staying in this phase for two weeks before moving to Phase Two:

Day One
Breakfast
Green Super Smoothie, page 66
Scrambled eggs
Cup of tea

Midmorning snack
Piece of fruit

Lunch
Lima Bean Winter Soup, page 86
Turkey sandwich with lettuce and tomato

Afternoon snack
Baby carrots and Chia Hummus, page 90

Dinner
Chia Chipotle Bean Burger, page 107
Sautéed spinach

Day Two
Breakfast
Basic Chia Protein Shake, page 67
2 links turkey sausage

Midmorning snack
Piece of fruit

Lunch
Power Wrap, pages 88–89
Cup of tomato soup

PROTEIN PACKED

Chia seeds contain about 20 percent protein, more than many other grains such as wheat and rice. Chia seeds also contain strontium, which helps our bodies assimilate protein and produce high energy.

Afternoon snack
Baby carrots or jicama slices with
    guacamole

Dinner
Chia Caesar Salad, pages 108–109
Mulligatawny Chia Soup, page 88

Day Three
Breakfast
1 cup low-sodium tomato
    juice, V8, or other vegetable juice
Chia Frittata, page 80

Midmorning snack
Raw veggie strips

Lunch
Chia Salad Sandwich, 90
Piece of fruit

Afternoon snack
1 cup air-popped popcorn

Dinner
2-ounce portion broiled salmon
½ cup brown rice
Green salad with vinaigrette

Day Four

Breakfast
1 cup low-sodium tomato juice, V8, or
    other vegetable juice
Chia-Oat Porridge, page 82

Midmorning snack
Apple slices with peanut butter

Lunch
Chia Rice Salad, page 92
Piece of fruit

Afternoon snack
1 ounce cashews

Dinner
1 cup vegetarian chili
Corn tortillas

Day Five

Breakfast
1 cup low-sodium tomato juice, V8, or
    other vegetable juice
Scrambled Chia Eggs, page 80

Midmorning snack
Piece of fruit

Lunch
Fast Soup, page 85
Chia Fruit Salad, page 94

Afternoon snack
Carrot sticks with Chia Hummus, page 90

Dinner
Black bean burger
Sautéed greens

DID YOU KNOW?

Chia has eight times more of the antioxidant and anti-inflammatory omega-3 fatty acid than salmon. You would have to eat 790 grams (about 1¾ pounds) of Atlantic salmon to get the same amount of omega-3 fatty acids contained in 100 grams (about 9 tablespoons) of chia.

Day Six

Breakfast
Green Super Smoothie, page 66
Oatmeal

Midmorning snack
Piece of fruit

Lunch
Large green salad with ½ cup chicken
Carrot sticks

Afternoon snack
1 ounce mixed nuts

Dinner
Beef stew

BLOOD SUGAR STABILIZER

A 2007 study published in *Diabetes Care* followed 20 people with Type 2 diabetes. Subjects were divided into two groups: A chia group and a wheat bran group. For 12 weeks, subjects took 37 grams of either chia or wheat bran. At the end of the study, those who took chia reduced systolic blood pressure and inflammation. And while they did not lose large amounts of weight, it was shown that they had more stable blood sugar levels than the control group. One common cause of food cravings is erratic blood glucose levels. By stabilizing these levels, there is the potential to ward off cravings, a side effect many chia consumers report.

Day Seven

Breakfast
Basic Chia Protein Shake, page 67
Piece of fruit

Midmorning snack
Baby carrots

Lunch
Chicken breast sandwich with lettuce and
    tomato
Piece of fruit

Afternoon snack
Jicama slices with guacamole

Dinner
Meatloaf
Green salad with Zippy Dressing,
    page 94

In some ways I do see chia as a miracle. It helps me to be satisfied with less food, helps keep me full longer so I don't want to snack as much as I used to, and it gives me more energy to exercise. None of these are extreme, "out there" ways to lose weight, but put together they've helped me to lose 18 pounds in a little under five months without going crazy or trying too hard.

—JANET CISCO,
Las Vegas, NV

OPTIONAL ONE-WEEK MENU, PHASE TWO:

In this phase, your body is comfortable with chia so it's a great time to add more. You'll see an increase in benefits as well as experiencing greater satiety at mealtime. Plan on being in Phase Two for a month before moving onto Phase Three.

Day One
Breakfast
Green Super Smoothie,
    page 66
½ cup oatmeal
Cup of tea

Midmorning snack
Piece of fruit

Lunch
Lima Bean Winter Soup, page 86
Small turkey sandwich with
    lettuce and tomato slices

Afternoon snack
Baby carrots and hummus

Dinner
Chia Chipotle Bean Burger, page 107
Sautéed spinach

Day Two
Breakfast
Basic Chia Protein Shake, page 67
Piece of fruit

Midmorning snack
Carrot and celery sticks with peanut butter

Lunch
Power Wrap, pages 88–89
Piece of fruit

Afternoon snack
Baby carrots or jicama slices with Chia
    Guacamole, page 101

Dinner
Chia Caesar Salad, pages 108–
    109

Day Three
Breakfast
1 cup low-sodium tomato juice,
    V8, or other vegetable juice
Chia Frittata, page 80

Midmorning snack
Veggie strips

Lunch
Chia Salad Sandwich, page 90
Piece of fruit

Afternoon snack
1 ounce roasted pumpkin seeds

Dinner
2-ounce portion broiled salmon
Mexican Grain Pilaf, pages 91–92
Green salad with Zippy Dressing,
    page 94

Day Four

Breakfast
1 cup low-sodium tomato juice, V8,
    or other vegetable juice
Chia-Oat Porridge, page 82

Midmorning snack
Piece of fruit

Lunch
Chia Rice Salad with added ½ cup of black
    beans, page 92

Afternoon snack
Raw veggie strips

Dinner
Chia Vegetarian Chili, page 103
Corn tortillas

Day Five

Breakfast
1 cup low-sodium tomato juice, V8,
    or other vegetable juice
Scrambled Chia Eggs, page 80

Midmorning snack
Piece of fruit

Lunch
Fast Soup, page 85
Green salad with ½ cup of chicken, turkey
    or ham

Afternoon snack
1 ounce raw almonds

Dinner
Chia Cottage Pie, page 104
Green salad

Day Six

Breakfast
Green Super Smoothie, page 66
Scrambled eggs

Midmorning snack
Piece of fruit

Lunch
Small turkey sandwich with lettuce and
    tomato
Mulligatawny Chia Soup, page 88

Afternoon snack
Celery with almond butter

Dinner
Chia Quesadilla with Chia Guacamole,
    pages 100–101
Grilled vegetables

DYS-WHAT?

Many studies on chia have found that it helps prevent or treat dyslipidemia. This word may sound unfamiliar, but it has a very clear meaning: Abnormal cholesterol levels, typically high cholesterol (also known as high blood cholesterol level).

DR. OZ ON CHIA

"Chia Pets may have no apparent purpose, but chia seed? Now, that's something to get excited about. Chia—a harvested, unprocessed, nutty-tasting, nutrient-dense whole grain with omega-3 fatty acids—has among the highest antioxidant activity of any whole food, outdistancing even fresh blueberries. One study showed that 30 grams of chia seed taken with bread decreased the sharp blood sugar spike seen an hour after eating. Another study showed that chia lowers blood pressure and the risk of heart problems. My recommendation: two daily doses of about 20 grams (about two tablespoons) of seeds each."

—DR. MEHMET OZ, *You: Staying Young* (Free Press, 2007)

Day Seven

Breakfast
Basic Chia Protein Shake, page 67
Piece of fruit

Midmorning snack
Carrots and Chia Hummus, page 90

Lunch
Chia Faux Enchiladas, page 106

Afternoon snack
Piece of fruit

Dinner
Chia Meatloaf, page 102
Sautéed broccoli

My husband's running partner recommended he take chia last year when he was gearing up for the NYC Marathon. I watched how much healthier he looked. His hair seemed fuller, his skin looked better, he seemed more even-tempered. So I began using chia, too. I stir it into my morning yogurt or oatmeal. People have commented on how young I look. I absolutely see a change in my skin and hair, and my eyes seem brighter, too. What I wasn't expecting is to lose some weight. I lost six pounds the first month I used it. I think because it filled me up and made me feel full longer, so I wasn't as tempted to snack as much as I used to.

—RITA MINARDI, Stamford, CT

OPTIONAL ONE-WEEK MENU,
PHASE THREE:

In Phase Three, you'll reach the amount of chia that researchers have found best supports weight loss and maintenance. You'll see an increase in benefits as well as greater satiety at mealtime. Plan on staying in Phase Three until you reach your goal weight.

Day One
Breakfast
Green Super Smoothie, page 66
Chia French Toast, page 79
Cup of tea

Midmorning snack
Chia Fresca, page 65
Piece of fruit

Lunch
Lima Bean Winter Soup, page 86
Nut Butter & Jelly Sandwich, page 80

Afternoon snack
Baby carrots and Chia Hummus, page 90

Dinner
Chia Chipotle Bean Burger, page 107
Sautéed spinach

Day Two
Breakfast
Basic Chia Protein Shake, page 67
Aussie-Style Broiled Tomato with Chia, page 84

Midmorning snack
Spicy Green Chocolate Shake, page 69

Lunch
Power Wrap, pages 88–89
Piece of fruit

Afternoon snack
Baby carrots or jicama slices with Chia Seed Guacamole, page 101

Dinner
Chia Caesar Salad, pages 108–109
Mulligatawny Chia Soup, page 88

Day Three
Breakfast
1 cup low-sodium tomato juice, V8, or other vegetable juice
Chia Frittata, page 80

Midmorning snack
Chia Fresca, page 65
Protein Muffin, pages 72–73

Lunch
Chia Salad Sandwich, 90
Chia Fruit Salad, page 94

Afternoon snack
Protein Bites, pages 95–96

Dinner
2-ounce portion broiled salmon
Mexican Grain Pilaf, pages 91–92
Green salad with Zippy Dressing, page 94

Day Four

Breakfast
1 cup low-sodium tomato juice, V8,
 or other vegetable juice
Chia-Oat Porridge, page 82

Midmorning snack
Chia Fresca, page 65
Chia Seed Muffin, page 71

Lunch
Chia Rice Salad, page 92
Piece of fruit

Afternoon snack
Moroccan Carrot Salad, page 93

Dinner
Chia Vegetarian Chili, page 103
Chia Cornbread, page 73

Day Five

Breakfast
1 cup low-sodium tomato juice, V8,
 or other vegetable juice
Scrambled Chia Eggs, page 80

Midmorning snack
Chia Fresca, page 65
Piece of fruit

Lunch
Fast Soup, page 85
Chia Fruit Salad, page 94

Afternoon snack
Almond Delight, page 66

Dinner
Chia Cottage Pie, page 104
Green Salad with Chia Sunshine Sauce,
 page 94

WHAT'S AN ANTIOXIDANT?

To understand antioxidants, it's important to first understand oxidants. Oxidation is a chemical reaction that transfers electrons or hydrogen from a substance to an oxidizing agent. Oxidation reactions can produce free radicals, or oxidants. In turn, these radicals can start chain reactions. When a chain reaction occurs in a cell, it can cause damage or death to the cell. An antioxidant is a molecule capable of inhibiting the oxidation of other molecules.

The easiest place to get these protective molecules is from plant food. Chia, the black seed in particular, is a rich, powerful source of antioxidants. Bright- and dark-colored fruits and vegetables are also rich in these powerful nutrients. Eating numerous servings daily of antioxidant-heavy food is one of the most effective ways to maintain wellness.

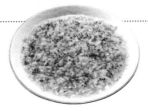

Day Six
Breakfast
Green Super Smoothie, page 66
Chia-Oat Porridge, page 82

Midmorning snack
Chia Fresca, page 65
Piece of fruit

Lunch
Large Green Salad with ½ cup chicken
    and Chia Sunshine Sauce, page 94
One slice Pumpkin Bread, page 75

Afternoon snack
Ginger Pear Eggnog Smoothie, page 68

Dinner
Creamy Mushroom-Cashew Soup, pages 86–87
Chia Quesadilla with Chia Guacamole,
    pages 100–101

Day Seven
Breakfast
Basic Chia Protein Shake, page 67
Piece of fruit

Midmorning snack
Chia Snack Bar, page 76

Lunch
Chia Faux Enchiladas, page 106

Afternoon snack
Citrus Julius, page 67

Dinner
Chia Meatloaf, page 102
Green salad with Zippy Dressing, page 94

A DIETER'S BEST FRIEND

Eating fiber helps create a feeling of fullness and satiety that takes the edge off hunger, which makes it less likely you'll turn to candy bars, cookies, chips or other packaged junk food to satisfy food cravings.

Fortunately, chia is loaded with fiber, both the soluble kind (which swells in water) and the insoluble kind (which doesn't). Just one tablespoon—12 grams—of chia boasts 5,000 mg of total fiber, the same amount of fiber as in:

- 10 cups of Corn Flakes cereal
- 10 slices white sandwich bread
- 1 ¼ cups of Kellogg's All Bran cereal
- An entire large cantaloupe
- 1 ¼ cup cooked oatmeal
- 2 ½ cups cooked white rice
- 1 ½ cup cooked carrots
- 2 ½ medium bananas
- 4 cups popcorn
- About 3 medium tomatoes

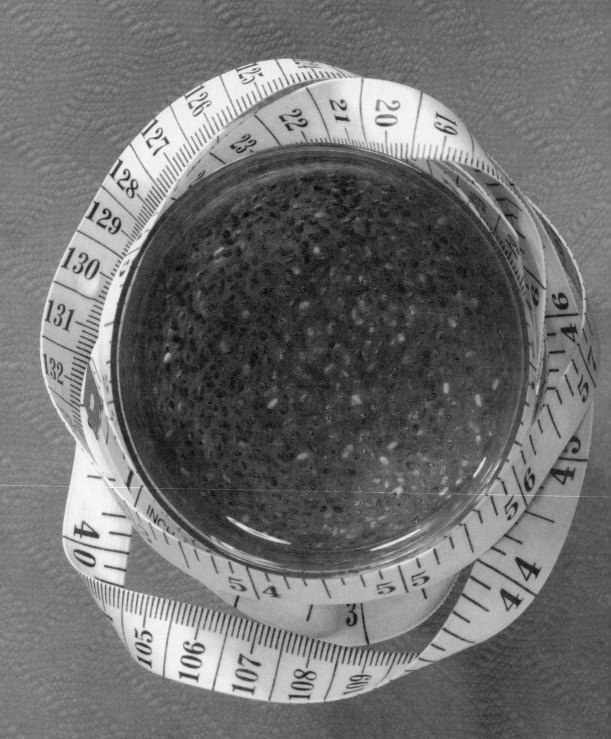

CHAPTER 3

CHIA AND WEIGHT MAINTENANCE

Anyone who has lost weight can tell you that losing weight is difficult, but keeping lost weight off is even more difficult. Fortunately, chia can help with this.

The maintenance plan in this chapter is for those of you who enjoy your current weight. It's also perfect for individuals who have gone through the phases outlined in Chapter Two and Chapter Four and want to stay healthy, fit, and motivated in order to maintain their good health.

THE MAINTENANCE PHASE

In this phase, you'll continue to consume the 45 grams of chia that researchers have found best supports weight loss and maintenance. For every step below, you can sprinkle chia onto your food or stir it into your food. If preferred, you could also mix it into a small glass of water or juice and drink it. You'll see an increase in benefits as well as greater satiety at mealtime. You can use this guide with your favorite healthy foods or diet program menus (such as Weight Watchers, Jenny Craig, South Beach Diet, etc.):

• **Breakfast:** 1 tablespoon whole chia seed or milled chia.
• **Midmorning snack:** ½ tablespoon whole chia seed or milled chia.
• **Lunch:** 1 tablespoon whole chia seed or milled chia.
• **Afternoon snack:** ½ tablespoon whole chia seed or milled chia.
• **Dinner:** 1 tablespoon whole chia seed or milled chia.

My grandmother used to make us agua fresca almost every day in the summer. I never thought much about this. But when Stephanie, my health coach, suggested I begin drinking agua fresca each afternoon to help combat the 3:00 pm fatigue that would wash over me, I listened: My grandmother used to always call this a "pick me up". After consuming chia, not only did I have the stamina to get through my day, I quickly found that I had stopped wanting sweet snacks in the afternoon. Soon I felt so healthy and full of energy, that I began taking a midday walk. I'm happy to say I have I lost 11 pounds in just over two months.
— MARIA RODRIGUEZ, Mexico City, Mexico

OPTIONAL MAINTENANCE MENUS

In this phase when you've reached the amount of chia consumption that best supports weight loss and maintenance, you'll continue to see an increase in benefits as well as experiencing greater satiety at mealtime.

Day One

Breakfast
Green Super Smoothie, page 66
Chia Breakfast Polenta, page 106
Cup of tea

Midmorning snack
Chia Fresca, page 65
Piece of fruit

Lunch
Lima Bean Winter Soup, page 86
Nut Butter & Jelly Sandwich, page 80

Afternoon snack
Baby carrots and Chia Hummus, page 90

Dinner
Chia Chipotle Bean Burger, page 107
Sautéed spinach

Day Two

Breakfast
Basic Chia Protein Shake, page 67
Aussie-Style Broiled Tomato with Chia, page 84

Midmorning snack
Spicy Green Chocolate Shake, page 69

Lunch
Power Wrap, pages 88–89
Piece of fruit

Afternoon snack
Baby carrots or jicama slices with Chia Seed Guacamole, page 101

Dinner
Chia Caesar Salad, pages 108–109
Mulligatawny Chia Soup, page 88

Day Three

Breakfast
1 cup low-sodium tomato juice, V8, or other vegetable juice
Chia Frittata, page 80

Midmorning snack
Chia Fresca, page 65
Protein Muffin, pages 72–73

JOINT SOOTHER

Many people with arthritis and other joint disorders report reduced pain and inflammation after a few weeks of taking chia seeds. The high concentration of omega-3 fatty acids in chia helps to "lubricate" joints and keep them supple. Additionally, omega-3 fatty acids are converted into prostaglandins, which are known to have both pain relieving and anti-inflammatory effects.

Lunch
Chia Salad Sandwich, 90
Chia Fruit Salad, page 94

Afternoon snack
Protein Bites, pages 95–96

Dinner
2-ounce portion broiled salmon
Mexican Grain Pilaf, pages 91–92
Green salad with Zippy Dressing, page 94

Day Four
Breakfast
1 cup low-sodium tomato juice, V8,
    or other vegetable juice
Chia-Oat Porridge, page 82

Midmorning snack
Chia Fresca, page 65
Chia Seed Muffin, page 71

Lunch
Chia Rice Salad, page 92

Piece of fruit

Afternoon snack
Moroccan Carrot Salad, page 93

Dinner
Chia Vegetarian Chili, page 103
Chia Cornbread, page 73

Day Five
Breakfast
1 cup low-sodium tomato juice, V8,
    or other vegetable juice
Scrambled Chia Eggs, page 80

Midmorning snack
Chia Fresca, page 65
Piece of fruit

Lunch
Fast Soup, page 85
Chia Fruit Salad, page 94

Afternoon snack
Almond Delight, page 66

Dinner
Chia Polenta with White Beans, page 105
Green salad with Chia Sunshine Sauce,
  page 94

Day Six
Breakfast
Green Super Smoothie, page 66
Chia-Oat Porridge, page 82

Midmorning snack
Chia Fresca, page 65

Piece of fruit

Lunch
Large green salad with ½ cup chicken and
  Chia Sunshine Sauce, page 94
One slice Pumpkin Bread, page 75

Afternoon snack
Ginger Pear Eggnog Smoothie, page 68

Dinner
Creamy Mushroom-Cashew Soup, pages 86–87
Chia Quesadilla with Chia Guacamole,
  pages 100–101

SEEDS THAT ACT LIKE GRAINS

A whole-food diet rich in non-cereal grains (such as "grain-like" seeds) is one of the best ways to lose weight. It's also the best way to provide your body with the nutrients and fiber it needs to be healthy and run efficiently. Here are a few grain-like seeds that perfectly complement chia. Give them a try:

• **Amaranth:** Like chia, amaranth is a seed. Also like chia, amaranth was an Aztec favorite. And lastly, like chia, amaranth is loaded with protein (8 grams per ¼ cup), fiber (7 grams per ¼ cup), iron (20 percent of the daily requirement in a ¼ cup) and a full-range of amino acids.

• **Quinoa** is technically a seed, not a grain. Another surprise: It's related to spinach and Swiss chard. Cultivated in the Andean mountain regions of Peru, Chile, and Bolivia for over 5,000 years, quinoa is rich in minerals, fiber, protein, and amino acids, and has long been a staple food in the diet of native Americans. The Incas considered it a sacred food and referred to it as the "mother seed."

• **Millet** is a seed that is rich in magnesium, a mineral that acts as a co-factor for more than 300 enzymes, including enzymes involved in the body's use of glucose and insulin secretion.

• **Buckwheat** is related to sorrel and rhubarb. Rich in phytonutrients, such as flavonoids, as well as minerals, buckwheat's strong flavor is much prized by some and is a staple in Eastern European cooking.

I originally began taking chia seven months ago to lower my blood pressure—I was hoping to cut down on my medication or get rid of it entirely. I have cut down on the medication, which I am very happy about. What was unexpected was weight loss. I've lost 13 pounds in the time I've been on it. I just don't have the desire to eat between meals like I used to. I also find it easier to exercise each day. Before, I'd want to quit after 20 minutes. I'd have a stitch in my side, or get thirsty, or have a muscle cramp or just get tired. Now, I can go for 30 to 45 minutes—even an hour—without quitting. So I am also getting a lot more exercise than I used to.

—JAMES SALTZER, San Diego, CA

Day Seven

Breakfast
Basic Chia Protein Shake, page 67
Piece of fruit

Midmorning snack
Chia Snack Bar, page 76

Lunch
Chia Faux Enchiladas, page 106

Afternoon snack
Citrus Julius, page 67

Dinner
Chia Meatballs,
  page 103
½ cup quinoa
Green salad
  with Zippy
  Dressing, page 94

DAILY MAINTENANCE WORKOUT

This workout is just as adaptable to your likes, needs, and abilities as the workouts featured in Chapter 4. Change things up and experiment with different components of the program. Be sure to give yourself several "low impact days" a week, to give your muscles a chance to regenerate.

- **Stretching:** Aim for 10 minutes of total body stretching a day. Although you can choose whatever stretches you want—from formal yoga moves to simply raising your arms over your head—be mindful of the many different muscles in the body so you can find stretches that work everything from your feet to your gluteus maximus to your shoulders to your neck.
- **Low-Impact Aerobics Three Times Per Week:** Go for 30 to 45 minutes of sustained

low-impact aerobics. This can be as simple as taking a brisk walk, getting on an exercise bike, or hitting the lap lane at your local pool. As you get stronger, try harder moves, such as going up and down stairs, walking up hills, strapping on wrist or ankle weights, or standing up as you cycle. Use your common sense, but don't be afraid to push yourself a bit.

- **High-Impact Aerobics Four Times Per Week:** Aim for 45 or more minutes of sustained high-impact aerobics. Your choice—do what you love and what works for you on a particular day. Suggestions include outdoor or indoor running, an aerobic dance or kickboxing class, or rebounding on a trampoline. Limiting high-impact aerobics to three times per week will allow your muscles and tendons to get strong gradually, which will help prevent injury. It also gives the heart and lungs time to get used to more intense exercise.

- **Strength Training:** Aim for ten minutes of *light* strength training three times a week on Low-Impact Aerobics Days only. This will give muscles a chance to recoup. This is another chance for you to choose the moves you like: Grab a pair of 2.5-pound hand weights and do bicep curls, squats, toe raises, and more. Or, hop on to a resistance machine. If you don't want to use weights, use your own body's resistance, by doing old-fashioned pushups, sit-ups, leg lifts, and anything else you may remember from high school gym class.

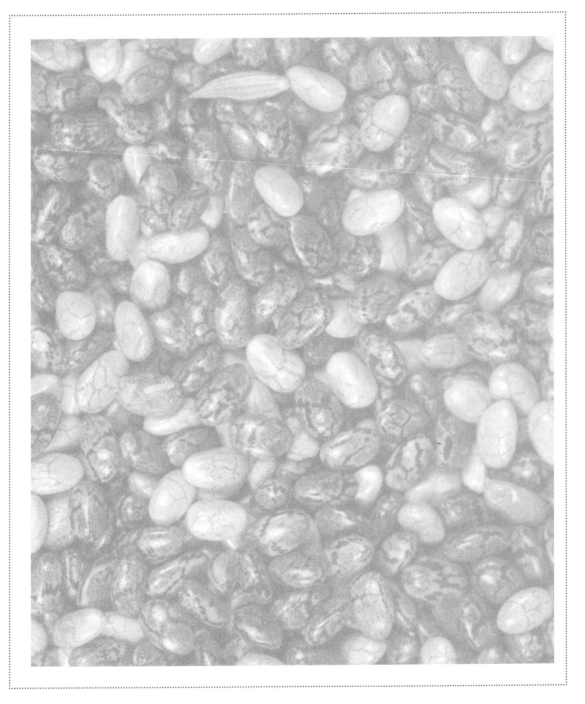

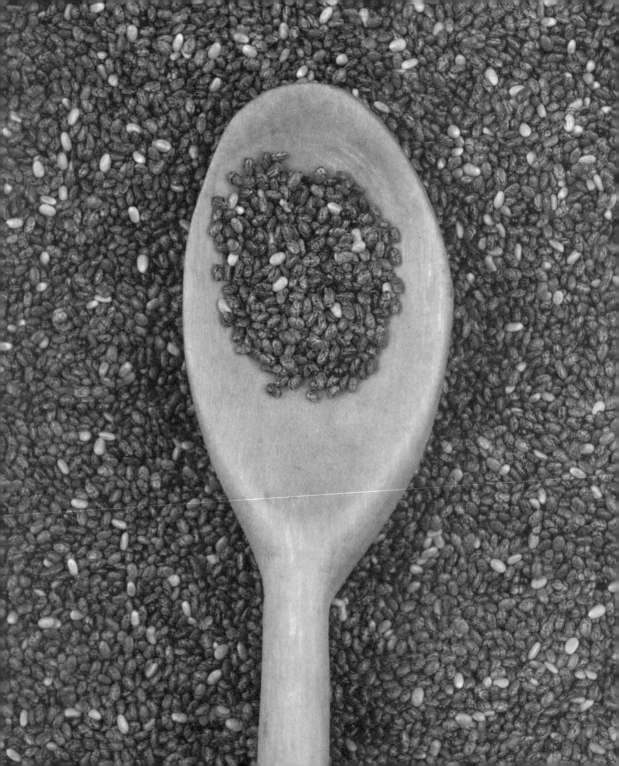

CHAPTER 4

THE CHIA EXERCISE, ENDURANCE, AND ENERGY PLAN

An exercise plan is an essential part of being healthy. You can eat all the chia in the world, but if you don't move your body, you won't have true health or be able to live up to your body's potential. Research backs this up:

- A 2011 study performed at the Fred Hutchinson Cancer Research Center in Seattle followed 439 sedentary postmenopausal women ages 50 to 75 who ranged from moderately overweight to obese, for an entire year. A quarter of the group did nothing, a quarter of the group exercised 45 minutes a day (moderate-to-vigorous aerobic exercise five days a week), a quarter of the group limited their calorie intake (1,200 to 2,000 calories a day, depending on starting weight, with fewer than 30 percent of the daily calories coming from fat), and a quarter of the group exercised *and* limited their calorie intake.

  The findings? The group that did nothing lost less than a pound during the study. The group that only exercised lost on average 2.4 percent of their starting weight, with an average weight loss of 4.4 pounds. The group that only dieted shed about 8.5 percent of their starting weight for an average of 15.8 pounds each. The group that both dieted and exercised did the best, shedding an average of 10.8 percent of their starting weight for an average of 19.8 pounds per person.

- In a 2006 study, University of Minnesota researchers found that for men, exercise alone could cause weight loss. Women, however, lost weight only when they decreased the number of high-fat packaged snack foods, dairy, and meat they ate by five to ten servings a week. Exercise helped speed and maintain weight loss in women, but did not work alone to help women reach their goal weights. Why? No one has yet figured this out.

- A 2006 study at the University of Westminster in London found that while dieting alone could help people lose weight it did not help a dieter to shed fat. A combination of dieting and exercise was needed to lose weight and replace fat with lean muscle. (Incidentally, a pound of fat takes up a whole lot more room than a pound of muscle, which explains why unfit people are a lot larger than fit people who weigh the same.)

GET READY TO MOVE

Human bodies were designed to move, which is why exercise makes good sense. Regular movement not only helps you shed weight faster and keep it off more successfully, it builds muscle, which helps create a leaner-looking, more fit body. And exercise has a host of health benefits, too, from lowering the risks of cancer and cardiovascular disease to boosting the immune system, squelching fatigue, aiding digestion, and creating a calmer nervous system.

If you've been adding chia to your diet—and now's the perfect time to begin experimenting with chia if you haven't yet—you may find that exercise feels easier than you expected. That's because chia actually helps the body exercise more and exercise more intensely. Here's how it works:

- Chia is hydrophilic and can absorb between nine and 12 times its weight in water. This means that chia increases body hydration, which is especially beneficial for athletes who need to remain hydrated during long races and endurance activities. Being well-hydrated means less fatigue and muscle cramping during workouts.
- The Aztecs used chia to help protect and heal joints. Chia is believed to decrease recovery time and fatigue in cardiovascular workouts by encouraging muscle tissue repair. Why? Omega-3 fatty acids and antioxidants, which are both found in chia, have been shown to reduce inflammation; hence they can help protect joints.
- Chia's moisture-retaining quality, plus its high potassium content, helps protect exercisers against electrolyte loss.

MIDDLE-AGE TRIUMPH

In 1997, Nike sponsored a 100-mile run in Colorado. Known as the Leadville Trail 100 Ultramarathon, the route is run at elevations higher than 10,000 feet. Twice, the course travels over the 12,600-foot Hope Pass. The grueling test was enough to make the youngest, fittest, best-outfitted professional marathoners blanch. Imagine what it would have felt like being a 50+ man running in sandals!

But that's just who ended up winning the race. Cirildo Chacarito, a 52-year-old Tarahumaran from a village near Chihuahua, Mexico, won the contest wearing homemade sandals fashioned of leather, used truck tires, and nails. Coming in second and fifth were his tribesmen Victoriano Churo and Manuel Luna. Chacarito completed the feat in 19 hours, 37 minutes, and 3 seconds. Instead of stopping at the aid stations lining the course, the men consumed the chia they brought from home, which they insisted helped them in their win.

THE MOVES

Before you start any fitness plan it's helpful to be familiar with four basic types of exercise in order to make the best fitness choices for yourself:

FLEXIBILITY WORK

Also known as stretching, flexibility work is essential to keeping your body supple, limber, and, yes, flexible. Have you ever noticed that one of the most common signs of aging is a shortened range of motion? In other words, humans tend to lose their flexibility as they age. Their steps get shorter. They shuffle. Their arms lose their swing. Their necks, shoulders, and backs no longer bend when and where they want them to.

Flexibility is important because it gives us range of motion, allowing us to take long, youthful strides, letting us execute all kinds of exercise and strength-building moves without harm, and reducing the likelihood of falls and injuries. Flexibility is essential if you want a body that "goes with the flow" and bounces back easily from physical exertion. Stretching can be as simple as the moves your high school track basketball or football coach taught you, or something more involved, such as yoga or Pilates.

LOW-IMPACT CARDIO

Also called low-impact aerobic exercise, low-impact cardio exercise is steady, prolonged exercise that continues longer than 20 or 30 minutes—such as swimming, walking, cross-country skiing, stair climbing, cycling, skating, rowing, or anything else that literally has a low impact on your joints.

Low-impact cardio is fantastic for anyone who needs to ease into exercise, such as the obese, anyone who has joint problems, or highly-fit individuals who want to alternate between high- and low-impact exercise a few times a week. Typically, low-impact cardio doesn't burn as many calories per minute or produce as much sweat as high impact cardio, but it is a more body-friendly option for everyone.

HIGH-IMPACT CARDIO

Also known as high-impact aerobics, high-impact cardio kicks things up a notch. Running, jumping, aerobic dance, kickboxing, jump roping, and rebounding on a mini-trampoline are all examples of high-impact cardio. Great for burning calories quickly, strengthening the lungs and heart, making you sweat, and strengthening bones, high-impact aerobic exercise is great for just about everyone, except pregnant women,

> *I am an experienced ultra-distance runner and have worn a heart rate monitor for years. I've stored all the data on my computer and find it interesting to see how the maximum values have dropped over the years and how the amount of high-intensity work outs have decreased as well. It is also interesting to see how many miles and hours a week I have been running, including total ascent during the runs, and ambient temperatures during the runs. I am not saying everyone needs this information, but it can be useful for you to track your progress as you improve your conditioning. Many people also use a heart rate monitor during runs to limit their speed, heart rate, and more, since this is an excellent way to ensure you don't overdo it!*
>
> —DR. WAYNE COATES

the obese, and anyone with joint problems. Aim for 30 or more minutes of sustained movement at a time.

RUNNING FOOD

In his book *Born to Run* (Knopf, 2009), Christopher MacDougal writes about the Tarahumara peoples of Copper Canyon, in the southwestern part of Mexico. These people are famous for their endurance, as well as their love of ultra-distant runs (sometimes 100 miles or more). MacDougal even found 90-year-old Tarahumaras running. One of their many secrets? Chia. The Tarahumara roast the seed, then crush it into a powder and mix it with water to make a basic "sports gel," which many consume daily, as well as right before running.

STRENGTH TRAINING

Strength training is any exercise that builds your muscles, whether it is push-ups, sit-ups, bench presses, or exercises with dumbbells, wrist weights, or kettleballs, or a fancy resistance machine. Building muscle should be an important part of your fitness strategy.

Having more muscles creates a lean, healthy-looking body that burns calories efficiently and keeps you strong, which is important if you want enough energy to get through your daily activities without becoming fatigued. Muscles enhance physical endurance—making it less likely that you'll become winded after walking up a few flights of stairs or running after your toddler—and help you get things done, from lifting a chair, to opening a tightly-sealed jar.

THE RULES

Before you start moving, here are the ground rules: Check in with your healthcare provider if you haven't exercised in a while. Choose the correct exercise program for your fitness level (jumping to a higher level will only cause you pain—it's best to start easy and build up to more intense workouts).

First, commit to getting some movement every single day. Every. Single. Day. Post it in your calendar if you must. Schedule it in your electronic diary. Just make sure you do it daily. This is especially important if you are trying to burn calories and shed pounds.

A 2009 study at the University of Colorado School of Medicine found that exercisers didn't actually experience "afterburn"—that much-touted (and perhaps near-mythical) revving-up of the metabolism that some fitness pros claim continues for hours after exercise. For the study, researchers recruited several groups of people, some of whom were lean endurance athletes, while others were either sedentary and lean or sedentary and obese. Each of the subjects spent several 24-hour periods in a special laboratory room called a walk-in calorimeter that measures the number of calories a person

YOUR TARGET HEART RATE

Some fitness pros and exercise buffs like to talk about target heart rate. Your *maximum* heart rate is approximately 220 minus your age. If you are 30 years old, your maximum heart rate is 190 beats per minute (BPM).

Your *target* heart rate is roughly 50 to 85 percent of your maximum heart rate. This is the level at which your heart is beating with moderate to high intensity, and sustaining a workout at this pace strengthens the heart and lung muscles. Beginners should exercise in the 50 to 60 percent target heart rate zone. Intermediate or average exercisers should aim for 60 to 70 percent. Advanced athletes can train in the 75 to 85 percent zone. To track your heart rate during exercise, you can take your pulse or use a heart rate monitor.

While finding your heart rate is fun (if you like this sort of thing), it isn't necessary for most healthy people. Simply exercise for 30 or more minutes until you are pleasantly winded.

That said, many physicians have strong opinions about target heart rates for people who are obese or pregnant, or have respiratory conditions or a cardiovascular disease (such as high blood pressure). If you fall into one of these categories, talk to your healthcare provider before beginning any new exercise regimen.

burns, followed by another 24 hour-period that included an hour-long bout of stationary bicycling. Researchers found that none of the groups, including the athletes, experienced "afterburn" or "metabolism revving."

According to findings, it seems that exercise's calorie-burning benefits happen during exercise itself. Period. This likelihood is all the more reason to get some movement in every single day.

As you'll see in a bit, the workouts described here are flexible, mix-and-match programs, designed to allow you to do what you love in order to shape up and slim down. All you have to do is choose your own blend of stretching, aerobic, and strength activities on any given day. Feel free to do try new stretches, aerobic exercises, or new strength training moves every single day.

DAILY WORKOUT LEVEL I

For people who are new exercisers, obese, injured, have pre-existing conditions, and whose healthcare providers have suggested gentle options, this may be your life fitness plan (if your healthcare provider feels it's best for you). Otherwise, plan to spend two or more months at this daily workout level before moving up to Level II. Advancing too quickly can leave you injured and burnt out.

STRETCHING

Aim for five to ten minutes of total body stretching a day. Although you can choose the stretches you want—from formal yoga moves to simply raising your arms over your head— be mindful of the many different muscles in the body so you can find stretches that work everything from your feet to your gluteus maximus to your shoulders to your neck.

WHY YOU SHOULD CONSIDER RUNNING

If you haven't tried distance running, and want to, what are you waiting for? The American College of Sports Medicine Position Statement on Exercise states that individuals who run more than 50 miles per week had significantly greater increases in HDL cholesterol (the good kind) and significantly greater decreases in body fat, triglyceride levels, and the risk of coronary heart disease than individuals who ran less than 10 miles per week. In addition, the long-distance runners had it over the short-distance runners with a nearly 50 percent reduction in hypertension and more than a 50 percent reduction in the use of medications used to lower blood pressure or cholesterol levels. Note: Many studies find the same benefits are available to those who run the more doable 25 to 35 miles per week.

I am busy, overworked, and always on the go. Like most everyone else today, I began taking chia at the suggestion of my nutritionist. I was telling her how tired I would get each afternoon. So tired that there were times when I would literally shut my office door, put my head down on my desk, and take a nap. I knew I had to do something about this when my boss caught me sleeping one day. Hence, the chia. I now have a bag at my desk that I sprinkle onto my lunchtime salad. It has made an enormous difference in my energy level. I even have time after work to play soccer or basketball with my son.

—JAMES PETERS, Los Angeles, CA

LOW-IMPACT AEROBICS

Try for 20 to 30 minutes of sustained low-impact aerobics. This can be as simple as taking a brisk walk or jumping on an exercise bike. As you get stronger, try harder moves, such as going up and down stairs, walking up hills, strapping on wrist or ankle weights, or standing up as you cycle. Use your common sense, but don't be afraid to push yourself a bit.

This is another chance for you to choose the moves you like: Grab a pair of 2.5-pound hand weights and do bicep curls, squats, toe raises, and more. Or hop on to a resistance machine. If you don't want to use weights, use your own body's resistance by doing old-fashioned push-ups, sit-ups, leg lifts, and anything else you may remember from high school gym class.

STRENGTH TRAINING

Aim for five to ten minutes of *light* strength training each day, making sure not to do the same exercise two days in a row—muscles need a break to regenerate. Since you are not using large amounts of weight or strength training for long periods of time, you can work your muscles daily without worry.

YOGA VS. WALKING

While yoga is terrific exercise, most types are far from aerobic. For instance, a 150-pound person will burn 150 calories in an hour of doing regular yoga, compared to 311 calories for an hour of walking at 3 mph.

DAILY WORKOUT LEVEL II

For those who are graduating from Daily Workout Level I or who are already moderately fit, Daily Workout Level II is a little more challenging, yet every bit as creative as the other workouts featured here. Plan to spend two or more months on this level before moving up to Daily Workout Level III. Advancing too quickly can leave you injured and burnt out.

COLON CANCER AND EXERCISE

Researchers from Washington University and Harvard University reviewed 52 studies, from the last 25 years, which linked exercise and the incidence of colon cancer, a cancer that is diagnosed in over 100,000 Americans each year. Their findings? Individuals who exercised the most (5 to 6 hours per week) were 24 percent less likely to develop the disease than those who exercised the least (less than 30 minutes per week).

STRETCHING

Aim for ten minutes of total body stretching. Although you can choose whatever stretches you want—from formal yoga moves to simply raising your arms over your head—be mindful of the many different muscles in the body so you can find stretches that work everything from your feet to your gluteus maximus to your shoulders to your neck.

A stretching note from Dr. Coates: Be careful here not to overdo it, since cold muscles are more easily injured than warm muscles. If you feel you are able to go for a little run or brisk walk prior to stretching, this seems to work best. Also, you should conclude your daily routine with a bit of stretching, when your muscles are warm and flexible.

LOW-IMPACT AEROBICS FOUR TIMES PER WEEK

Go for 30 to 45 minutes of sustained low-impact aerobics. This can be as simple as taking a brisk walk, getting on an exercise bike,

I've been doing 5Ks for about six months now as a fun way to get some exercise. Before going on chia, however, I could never run an entire race. I would usually start walking at the 3.5 mark, which is exactly when I'd get an achy, fatigued, I'm-going-to-fall-o no achy feeling! Chia really does help me feel alive and energetic through an entire race.

—STEVE PHILPOT, Chicago, IL

EXERCISE FACTS

- Fit people tend to sweat more and sooner than unfit people. Their bodies are more efficient at cooling.
- Exercise boosts mental acuity by increasing blood circulation to the brain and increasing serotonin in the brain, which leads to improved mental clarity and processing speed.
- With moderate exercise, most individuals will lose about one quart (4 cups) of fluid per hour. One tablespoon of chia gel (see page 77) taken before exercise can reduce the amount of fluid you lose, but be sure to drink 16 ounces of water shortly after working out to ensure that you remain properly hydrated.
- If your workout clothes smell like ammonia after a workout, you're burning a lot of protein for fuel. Ammonia is a by-product of protein metabolism. This is not a good thing, since burning protein means you may be burning your muscle tissue for energy instead of carbohydrates or body fat.
- Exercise decreases the harmful effects of stress by calming the body and increasing feel-good neurotransmitters such as serotonin and melatonin.
- To determine if your scale is correct, set a dumbbell or a weight plate on it. If the numbers don't match, try another weight and see if it's off by the same amount. Adjust your scale accordingly.
- Because exercise releases endorphins into the body, a daily workout can be just what you need to help improve energy levels all day.
- In 1982, the most expensive running shoe on the market was the Nike Air Columbia at a stratospheric $64.99.
- Daily movement helps slow degenerative joint disease by strengthening bones, muscles, and tendons.
- The average exercise life of a running shoe is about 400 miles.
- Most folks who wear their running shoes around on a regular basis usually only get around 200 running miles out of the shoes!

or hitting the lap lane at your local pool. As you get stronger, try harder moves, such as going up and down stairs, walking up hills, strapping on wrist or ankle weights, or standing up as you cycle. Use your common sense, but don't be afraid to push yourself a bit.

I'm the mother of twin toddler boys. With broken sleep, hormonal issues, and the physical demands of caring for young children, it's normal to be tired as a mother. I was so tired by late morning each day that I felt I couldn't safely look after my children the way I needed to. Chia has really helped maintain my energy levels, making me a safer, calmer, and more fun parent. A good thing for the entire family and no more difficult than a couple spoonfuls mixed into my morning veggie juice.

—MISSY ROBERTS, Miami

HIGH-IMPACT AEROBICS THREE TIMES PER WEEK

Aim for 20 or 30 minutes of sustained high-impact aerobics. It's your choice—do what you love and what works for you on a particular day. Suggestions include outdoor or indoor running, an aerobic dance or kickboxing class, or rebounding on a trampoline. Limiting high-impact aerobics to three times per week will allow your muscles and tendons to get strong gradually, which will help prevent injury and also give your heart and lungs time to get used to more intense exercise.

STRENGTH TRAINING

Aim for five to 10 minutes of strength training each day, making sure not to do the same exercise two days in a row—muscles need a break to regenerate. Since you are not using large weight or strength training for long periods of time, you can work your muscles daily without worry.

This is another chance for you to choose the moves you like: Grab a pair of 2.5-pound hand weights and do bicep curls, squats, toe raises, and more. Or hop on to a resistance machine. If you don't want to use weights, use your own body's resistance, by doing old-fashioned push-ups, sit-ups, leg lifts, and anything else you may remember from high school gym class.

AN EVERYDAY HABIT

The Aztecs consumed chia every single day, in unleavened bread, porridge, and drinks. They used the oil on their skin, blended it into medicine, and used it for a type of communion or sacrament in their religious ceremonies. For the Aztecs, chia was not only a superfood, it was an everyday staple. With the continual consumption of chia—as well as other nutrient-dense foods such as amaranth and dried beans—the Aztecs were famed for their vigor, strength, and physical prowess.

DAILY WORKOUT LEVEL III

For those who are graduating from Daily Workout Level II, or who are already fit, Daily Workout Level III is the most challenging. It's just as adaptable to your likes and needs and abilities as the other workouts featured here. You can stay at this level, changing things up and experimenting with different components of the program. Be sure to give yourself several "low impact days" a week, to give muscles a chance to regenerate.

STRETCHING

Aim for ten minutes of total body stretching. Although you can choose whatever stretches you want—from formal yoga moves to simply raising your arms over your head—be mindful of the many different muscles in the body so you can find stretches that work everything from your feet to your gluteus maximus to your shoulders to your neck.

LOW-IMPACT AEROBICS THREE TIMES PER WEEK

Go for 30 to 45 minutes of sustained low-impact aerobics. This can be as simple as taking a brisk walk or getting on an exercise bike or hitting the lap lane at your local pool. As you get stronger, try harder moves, such as going up and down stairs, walking up hills, strapping on wrist or ankle weights, or standing up as you cycle. Use your common sense, but don't be afraid to push yourself a bit.

I am a fitness instructor and personal trainer, who is on the go all day, six days a week. I would literally conk out every day right before having to teach my 2:00 high impact aerobics class. I dreaded this part of the day and felt I wasn't energetic enough to motivate the class. At my fiancé's suggestion (he's a weight lifter), I began taking two tablespoons of chia mixed with water each day (one with breakfast one with lunch). After about five days on chia, I noticed I got through the class with ease. Working with my late afternoon private clients was also much easier. The endurance that chia gives me is good for me, good for my business. My only regret about chia is that I didn't discover it earlier!

—SHARI CONNORS, Cincinnati, OH

HIGH-IMPACT AEROBICS FOUR TIMES PER WEEK

Aim for 45 or more minutes of sustained high-impact aerobics. It's your choice—do what you love and what works for you on a particular day. Suggestions include outdoor or indoor running, an aerobic dance or kick-boxing class, or rebounding on a trampoline. Limiting high-impact aerobics to three times per week will allow your muscles and tendons to get strong gradually, which will help prevent injury. It also gives the heart and lungs time to get used to more intense exercise.

MORE EXERCISE FACTS

- Running one mile burns approximately 30 percent more calories than walking one mile, and that formulation remains true whether you run outdoors or on a treadmill.
- The record for running a mile backward is 6:02.35, by D. Joseph James of India on August 10, 2002.
- In a study on walking and cognitive function, researchers found that women who walked 1.5 hours per week had significantly better cognitive function and less cognitive decline than women who walked less than 40 minutes per week.
- Running shoes are excellent for a regular walking program.
- When walking at a moderate pace, a 150-pound man burns 100 calories per mile; a 200-pound man burns 133 calories per mile; and a 250-pound man burns 166 calories per mile.
- Running uphill burns 28 percent more fat than cycling uphill.
- The first company to charge $100 for a pair of shoes was New Balance, who introduced the now legendary 990 in 1983.
- When a shoe "breaks down" it's usually in the midsole and not the outsole that goes first.
- Human thigh bones are stronger than concrete.
- Women in the Nurse's Health Study (72,488 female nurses) who walked three hours or more per week reduced their risk of a heart attack or other coronary event by 35 percent compared with women who did not walk.
- Want to keep your ankles strong? Do not use running shoes for lateral activities like tennis, basketball, step aerobics, racquetball, or any other sport that causes you to pivot and cut from side to side. Instead, go for a "cross-trainer" or "court shoe."
- People with flat feet are more prone to ankle sprains than those who have normal arches. If you have high arches you are even less likely to sprain your ankle than people who have regular arches.

WHAT IS ISKIATE?

If you're a runner, you may have heard of iskiate, a nutritious, whole food, homemade sports drink, based on an ancient recipe for Aztec Chia Fresca, the ingredients of which are water, chia, sweetener, and lemon or lime-juice. Some companies today sell pre-made "iskiate" powder that can be mixed with water.

Some say the term iskiate comes from the Tarahumara Indians of Mexico's Copper Canyon, near Chihuahua. Famous for their hardiness and distance running, the Tarahumara are dedicated chia eaters, believing that it provides energy and aids endurance. But word sleuths among you, beware: There is no clear history of the word, which may have come from the Tarahumara or from some other source altogether.

STRENGTH TRAINING

Aim for 10 minutes of *light* strength training three times a week on Low-Impact Aerobics days only. This will give your muscles a chance to recoup. This is another chance for you to choose the moves you like: Grab a pair of 2.5-pound hand weights and do bicep curls, squats, toe raises and more. Or, hop on to a resistance machine. If you don't want to use weights, use your own body's resistance, by doing old-fashioned pushups, sit-ups, leg lifts, and anything else you may remember from high school gym class.

I'm a casual runner, who runs about 15 to 18 miles a week. I also cycle, walk, row, play tennis, and swim. I began taking chia nine months ago, when I noticed that my running partner began to run longer distances than me without getting winded. He said he'd started blending chia into his breakfast smoothies. I tried it, too. Within one week, I no longer felt fatigued and out of breath toward the end of my runs. I really notice a difference in my endurance and lung capacity when I take chia.
—JOEL COHEN, Atlanta, GA

My son is a competitive college swimmer. His coach suggested chia to the entire swim team. After hearing my son raving about the change in his performance and mood, I began taking chia every day, too. I'm not a competitive athlete by any measure, but I will tell you that I now can get through my kickboxing class without feeling as if I am going to die (or at least pass out)! Because I am exercising better, I am losing weight faster: 18 pounds after almost four months on chia.

—SHARON BAKER, Minneapolis, MN

WHEN TO EXERCISE: IS THERE A BEST TIME?

Most people would agree that the best time to exercise is the time you are most likely to stick with it, whenever that happens to be. That said, there have been studies showing that exercising at certain times bestows certain benefits:

- While researching the effects of exercise on blood pressure, Appalachian State University researcher Sr. Scott Collier found that individuals who exercised at 7:00 a.m. experienced a 10 percent reduction in blood pressure that carried through the remainder of the day, dipping down to a 25 percent decrease by night fall. They also had longer and more beneficial sleep cycles than when they exercised at other times during the day.
- Researchers studying sleep apnea have found that mid- to late afternoon is the best time to exercise if you suffer from sleep apnea and want a good night's sleep.
- Research from Northwestern University points to late afternoon being the best time to exercise, as strength and physical stamina is at its peak during those times, which lessens chances of injury. This has something to do with body temperature: it is theorized that exercise is most productive when body temperature is at its highest, which is typically between 2:00 and 6:00 p.m.
- A 2010 study in Belgium found the best time to exercise to burn fat was in the morning, before breakfast (perhaps after a spoonful of chia?). For six weeks, 28 men were fed a diet of 50 percent fat, with 30 percent more calories than the men's normal diet. One group did no exercise, one group exercised in the morning before eating, and the last group exercised later in the day after meals. Only the group that exercised before breakfast gained almost no weight and showed no signs of insulin resistance.

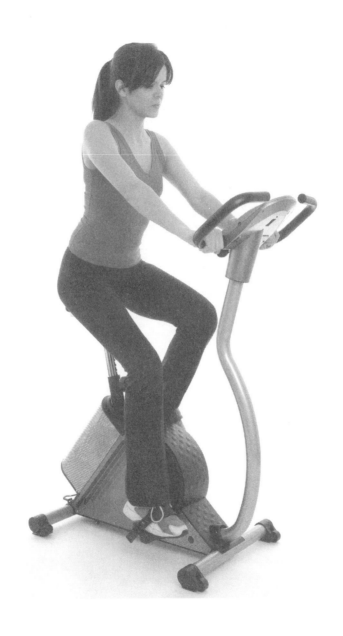

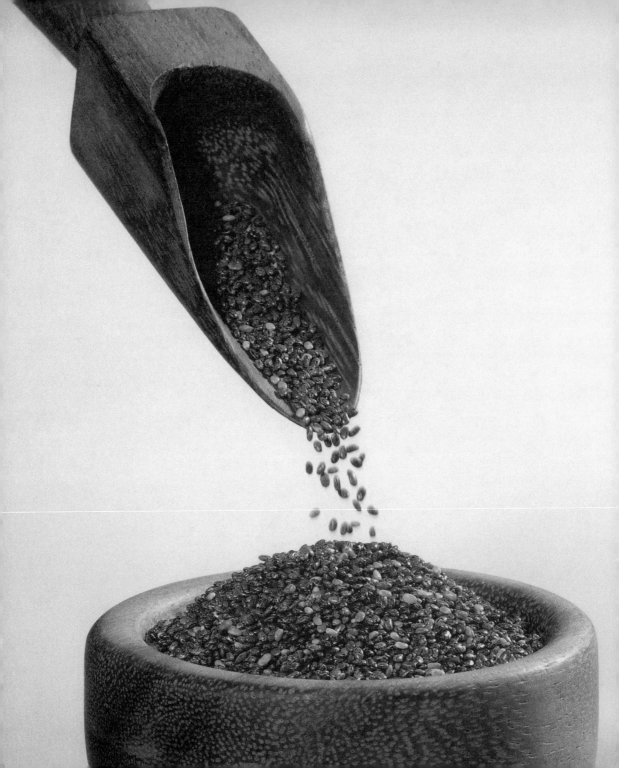

CHAPTER 5

COOKING, EATING, AND HEALING WITH CHIA

Chia is perfectly at home in the kitchen. It's easy to store, easy to use, and doesn't require grinders or other special equipment. Chia is versatile: it can be used at any temperature; it has a neutral taste; and the seeds possess a pleasant, almost nutty texture.

Chia's low-key personality is just as wonderful. Chia is the ultimate supporting player, quietly lending a high-impact dose of nutrients and fiber to the foods you already enjoy. This makes it ideal for all you "sneaky chefs" out there who are trying to get healthy foods into your fussy children's diet. As you'll see here, it's very easy to tuck chia is into a wide variety of recipes. Just scoop, sprinkle, and enjoy. The recipes below are perfect for anyone who's ready to maintain a healthy weight and create massive wellness. Bon appetit!

BEVERAGES

CHIA FRESCA
SERVES ONE

This ancient beverage has been used as an endurance booster by many of people living in Central America, as well as Mexico and the American Southwest. Refreshing and filling, Chia Fresca supplies a slow, steady supply of energy. It's a favorite of many distance runners who jokingly refer to Chia Fresca as "Home-Brewed Red Bull." For a change, swap in coconut water—it's a great way to add a quick dose of electrolytes to this refreshing beverage.

1 tablespoon chia seeds
8 to 10 ounces cool water (or coconut water)
  Juice of a half or whole lemon or lime
  (depending upon how tart you like things)
  Optional: Natural sweetener of your choice,
  to taste (sugar, honey, agave, brown rice
  syrup, Stevia, etc.)

1. Add chia seed to a glass of water, stirring until combined. Drink immediately if desired, or set aside for up to 10 minutes to allow the seed to form a gel.
2. Add lemon or lime juice and sweetener to the chia mixture, stirring until combined.
3. Drink immediately or let stand until mixture becomes gel-like.

GREEN SUPER SMOOTHIE

SERVES ONE

Green smoothies are all the rage. They are a great way to get a bold dose of veggies, fiber, and nutrients in a healthy, convenient, low-calorie way. Here, a tablespoon of chia seed creates an even more super-charged drink. This treat is best made in a high-powered blender. A Blendtec or Vitamix brand power blender is ideal.

1   tablespoon chia seeds
1½ cups pear juice, coconut water, water,
*   or a mixture*
3   romaine lettuce or kale leaves
1   small cucumber, peeled
*   Parsley sprigs*

1. Add all ingredients to a blender and liquefy using the most powerful setting. Blend until smooth.
2. Drink immediately.

ALMOND DELIGHT

SERVES ONE

This slightly sweet, creamy drink is perfect to round out breakfast, but it also makes a great snack or a healthy dessert after dinner. The recipe is versatile—have fun customizing it by using different milks, nut butters, and even fruits.

1   tablespoon chia seeds
1½ cup unsweetened almond milk
1   tablespoon almond butter
Optional: a dash of almond or vanilla extract
Optional: a small amount of natural sweetener
*   (such as honey, brown rice syrup, agave,*
*   Stevia, etc.)*

1. Add all ingredients to a blender and liquefy using the most powerful setting. Blend until smooth.
2. Drink immediately.

BASIC CHIA PROTEIN SHAKE
SERVES ONE

This easy recipe is based on one by the talented Jackie Rafter, holistic nutritionist and founder of LivLong Inc, at **http://livlong.ca**. It's incredibly versatile, so feel free to add and subtract ingredients at will, and design a new creation each time you make it.

1   *tablespoon chia seeds*
1½ *cup liquid of choice (water, coconut water, juice, rice milk, etc.)*
½ to 1 *cup chopped raw vegetable of your choice (¼ cup of this can be fruit)*
1   *tablespoon coconut oil*
1   *scoop protein powder of choice (hemp, rice, whey, etc.)*
3 or 4 *ice cubes*
Optional: A dash of your favorite extract or spice (such as vanilla, cinnamon, or allspice), a tablespoon of nut butter, a half-tablespoon of cocoa, cocoa nibs, or carob, etc.
Optional: Small amount of natural sweetener (such as honey, brown rice syrup, agave, Stevia, etc.)

1. Add all ingredients to a blender and liquefy using the most powerful setting. Blend until smooth.
2. Drink immediately.

CITRUS JULIUS
SERVES ONE

Here's another delicious recipe from holistic nutritionist Jackie Rafter, who says, "If you didn't know better, you'd think someone just bought you a delicious Grapefruit Julius! It's incredibly refreshing and a wonderful liver tonic, too."

1   *tablespoon chia seeds*
1   *grapefruit, juiced*
2   *lemons or limes, juiced*
1   *cup cool water*
1   *inch piece fresh ginger root, peeled*
Optional: Dash cayenne
Optional: Stevia powder for sweetening

1. Add all ingredients to a blender and liquefy using the most powerful setting. Blend until smooth.
2. Drink immediately.

GINGER PEAR EGGNOG SMOOTHIE

SERVES ONE

This festive shake is decadent and quick, making it the perfect treat for action-packed holidays. The recipe comes, once again, from Jackie Rafter. Here's her take on this delicious concoction: "This shake almost tastes like Christmas eggnog—A wonderful way to start your day or a great pick-me-up before going out on the town."

1 *tablespoon chia seeds*
1 *large pear, peeled, cut in half, and core removed*
1½ *cups water*
1 *scoop vanilla protein powder (hemp, rice, or whey, etc.)*
½ *inch piece fresh ginger root, peeled*
½ *teaspoon cinnamon, or a mix of cinnamon, clove, and nutmeg*
Optional: Stevia to sweeten
3 or 4 ice cubes

1. Add all ingredients to a blender and liquefy using the most powerful setting. Blend until smooth.
2. Drink immediately.

SPICY GREEN CHOCOLATE SHAKE

SERVES ONE TO TWO

This delectable shake combines chocolate and veggies to create a powerful source of nutrients. "Plus, it's green, very alkalizing, full of minerals, and it's incredibly healthy," says its creator, Jackie Rafter. "If you're really brave, load up with ½ teaspoon of the cinnamon and double the raw ginger."

1   tablespoon chia seeds
2 or 3 tablespoons raw cacao powder or
      ¼ cup carob or cacao nibs
2   cups water
3   cups raw baby spinach
½   avocado, peeled
1 or 2 scoops chocolate or vanilla flavor
      protein powder (rice, hemp, or whey, etc.)
1   teaspoon ginger powder or 1-inch fresh
      ginger root, peeled
1   teaspoon cinnamon
8   ice cubes
      Stevia to taste
Optional: ¼ to ½ teaspoon spirulina or
      chlorophyll powder
Optional: 1 teaspoon lecithin powder

1. Add all ingredients to a blender and liquefy using the most powerful setting. Blend until smooth.
2. Drink immediately.

IT'S A KEEPER

Many whole foods—such as brown rice, flaxseed, and wheat germ—go rancid quickly or are prone to infestations by hungry pests. Not chia! Thanks to concentrated levels of antioxidants, chia resists spoilage, even when kept in a room temperature cupboard for two years!

FRUIT SLUSHY

SERVES ONE

This refreshing shake is a supercharged version of those fruit-flavored (neon-colored) Slurpee beverages found at quick marts throughout the United States. Quick, easy, and addictively delicious, this is a great, easy-to-make snack recipe for kids.

1   tablespoon chia seeds
1½   cup cool water, coconut water, or juice of
        choice (pear is especially nice and considerably
        lower on the glycemic index than apple, grape,
        and other juice favorites, meaning it won't
        cause a blood sugar spike after drinking)
½ to 1 cup frozen fruit of your choice (you
        can use a blend of different fruits or stick
        to one kind)

1. Add all ingredients to a blender and liquefy using the most powerful setting. Blend until smooth.
2. Drink immediately.

TROPICAL CHAMPAGNE PUNCH SMOOTHIE

SERVES 10 TO 20

This is for all of you who like to mix health and pleasure. Created by holistic nutritionist Jackie Rafter, this punch is a special-occasion treat that combines chia, fruit, and alcohol (though Rafter also loves it without the wine). It was "test-driven" on almost 50 people who would have never guessed it was as healthy as it was delicious. "Plus it's so simple and easy to make," says Rafter, who created the recipe for her mother's 75th birthday. "The chia seed is excellent not only for adding body, but also for absorbing alcohol."

3 tablespoons chia seeds
1 grapefruit, juiced
1 or 2 oranges, juiced
1 inch piece of fresh ginger root, peeled
1 banana, peeled
½ a mango, peeled and chopped
¼ fresh pineapple, peeled and chopped
2 to 3 cups cool water
  Stevia, to sweeten
1 bottle champagne or sparkling wine
  Generous amounts of ice

1. Add all ingredients, except wine and ice, to a blender and liquefy using the most powerful setting. Blend until smooth.
2. Pour into a punch bowl and add champagne.
3. Adjust sweetener if necessary.
4. Add ice.

HANGOVER CURE?

There are several underground reports that chia is used to prevent hangovers, or as a way to lessen the effect of a full-blown hangover. While we haven't tried this ourselves, it makes sense: Chia contains high levels of vitamins A, B complex, C, and E, as well as ferulates and many phytonutrients—all of which help the body get rid of unwanted toxins, and all of which are depleted by alcohol. Furthermore, chia is hydrating, so it can prevent and treat the dehydration caused by alcohol. To try this yourself, after a night of hitting the town, stir 1 tablespoon of chia into a glass of water before going to bed. Repeat upon waking if needed.

CHIA VS. SALBA

Anyone who has looked into chia has probably heard of Salba®. This is the trademarked name for white chia, which was originally planted and then produced in Peru. Tests have shown that white and black chia seeds have essentially the same composition, however, black seeds have higher levels of antioxidants.

BAKED TREATS

CHIA SEED MUFFINS
MAKES 12

Muffins are the quintessential grab-and-go breakfast treats, beloved of kids and adults alike. They're also a sweet snack—perfect for when you crave something sweet. These muffins are not only delicious, they're hearty and filling, thanks to the addition of chia.

1   *stick butter, softened*
¾   *cup raw or regular sugar*
2   *large eggs, lightly beaten*
¾   *cup plain yogurt, at room temperature*
1½ *teaspoons vanilla*
2   *cups whole wheat pastry flour or unbleached all-purpose four*
⅓   *cup chia seeds*
½   *teaspoon salt*
¼   *teaspoon baking soda*
Optional: Cinnamon sugar topping, made with 2 tablespoons sugar and ¼ teaspoon cinnamon

1. Preheat the oven to 375°F. Line a muffin tin with muffin papers or lightly grease a muffin tin.
2. In a large mixing bowl, cream the butter and sugar until light and fluffy. You can do this by hand, with a hand-held mixer, or in a stand mixer.
3. Blend in the eggs, yogurt, and vanilla.
4. In a separate bowl, combine the flour, chia seeds, salt, and baking soda.
5. Slowly add the dry ingredients to the creamed mixture and blend just until combined. Do not over mix.
6. Fill each muffin cup ⅔ full of batter.
7. Sprinkle with the cinnamon sugar, if using.
8. Bake until golden brown, 15 to 20 minutes. Allow the muffins to cool slightly before removing from the tin.

MILLED CHIA

Many of the recipes in this section call for milled chia. Though it sounds exotic, milled chia is nothing more than chia seeds that have been ground into meal so it can be used as a flour-like ingredient in baked goods.

To make your own milled chia, take as much chia as you'd like and grind it in a clean coffee mill, food processor, or high-speed blender (such as a Vitamix or Blendtec). Process the seed until it resembles sand in texture—you want a coarse flour. It keeps well, so go ahead and make extra so that you'll have milled chia handy for all your recipes.

GLUTEN-FREE CHIA MUFFINS
MAKES 2 DOZEN REGULAR OR
4 DOZEN MINI MUFFINS

Gluten is the protein found in wheat and wheat's cousins, including spelt, kamut, semolina, rye, and even barley. People with gluten intolerances and those with Celiac Sprue must avoid gluten. In this easy recipe, milled chia stands in for the standard wheat flour, illustrating just how simple it is to bake without wheat. **Note:** Try using your mini-muffin tins: The muffins bake up higher and lighter when made small.

1½ cups milled chia
2   teaspoons baking powder
½ teaspoon salt
1   large egg, lightly beaten
1   teaspoon vanilla
¼ cup oil or melted butter
½ cup milk (dairy, coconut, almond, rice, etc.)
¼ cup honey
Optional: 1 cup raisins, dried cranberries,
  chopped dried apricots, frozen blueberries,
  or chopped peaches

1. Preheat the oven to 350°F. Line two standard muffin tins or four mini muffin tins with muffin papers, or lightly greased muffin tins.
2. In a medium bowl, whisk together the chia, baking powder, and salt.
3. In a large bowl, mix together the egg, vanilla, oil, milk, and honey, combining thoroughly.
4. Add the dry ingredients to the liquid ingredients, then add the fruit, if using. Gently mix until just combined.
5. Fill each muffin cup ⅔ full of batter.
6. Bake in middle rack of the oven until golden brown, 20 to 25 minutes.
7. Cool in the tins for 5 minutes before removing.

BAKING WITHOUT GLUTEN
Gluten, the protein in wheat, gives baked goods structure and a soft, springy texture. If you've been told you have to give up gluten, you have options, one of them being chia. Just keep in mind that baked goods made without wheat may have either a heavier, moister texture, or a drier one, depending on the non-gluten flour you bake with.

PROTEIN MUFFINS
MAKES 12 MUFFINS

This muffin is great for anyone who needs a lot of protein—distance runners, power lifters, triathletes, pregnant women—as well as anyone who likes their muffins hearty. You can also pop them into your kids' lunch boxes or wrap up and tuck one into your bag for a mid-morning pick-up.

1   cup cooked black or white beans
⅓ cup milled chia
⅓ cup natural cocoa powder
½ cup raw or regular sugar

1 cup whole wheat pastry flour

1 teaspoon baking soda

1 teaspoon cinnamon

½ teaspoon ginger

½ teaspoon salt

1 cup shredded carrot (use about 2 medium-size carrots)

1 large egg, lightly beaten

⅓ cup virgin coconut oil, liquefied

1 teaspoon vanilla

1. Preheat oven to 350°F. Line a muffin tin with muffin papers, or lightly grease a muffin tin.

2. Puree the beans in a food processor or a high-power blender, such as a Vitamix or Blendtec. Set aside.

3. In a large bowl, whisk together the chia, cocoa, sugar, flour, baking soda, cinnamon, ginger, and salt.

4. In a separate bowl, combine the pureed beans, carrot, egg, coconut oil, and vanilla. Mix thoroughly.

5. Add the dry ingredients to the bean mixture, stirring gently until ingredients are combined.

6. Fill each muffin cup ⅔ full of batter.

7. Bake on the middle rack until a toothpick inserted in the muffins comes out clean, 15 to 20 minutes, checking often for doneness so as to not overcook.

8. Cool in the tins for 5 minutes before removing.

CHIA CORNBREAD
MAKES 6 TO 9 SERVINGS

Southern-style cornbread is the perfect accompaniment to sautéed greens, beans, chili, soups, and stews—and it makes a nourishing snack. This tasty, gluten-free version is made with fiber-rich, nutrient-dense chia.

3 tablespoons extra-virgin olive oil, virgin coconut oil, or other oil.

2 cups yellow or white cornmeal

1 teaspoon baking powder

1 tablespoon milled chia

½ teaspoon salt

1 large egg, beaten

1½ cups milk (dairy, buttermilk, rice milk, almond milk, coconut milk, etc.)

1. Preheat the oven to 375°F.

2. Pour the oil in a 9-inch cast-iron skillet or similar-sized glass baking dish and transfer to the preheating oven.

3. Whisk the cornmeal, baking powder, milled chia, and salt in a medium bowl until combined.

4. Add the egg and milk; stir until just combined.

5. Remove the pan from the oven and swirl the oil to coat the bottom and a little way up the sides. Very carefully pour the excess hot oil into the cornmeal mixture; stir until just combined.

6. Pour the batter into the hot pan. Bake until the bread is firm in the middle and lightly golden, about 20 minutes.

7. Let cool for 5 minutes before slicing. Serve warm.

BANANA BREAD

MAKES 6 TO 9 SERVINGS

Who doesn't love banana bread? Sweet, fruity, and satisfying, this homey treat is true comfort food. Here, it is revved up with chia, making it a healthy snack option.

5   *tablespoons butter (softened), plus more for greasing pan*
½   *cup raw or regular sugar*
2   *large eggs (or egg substitute equivalent), at room temperature*
1½ *cups all-purpose flour*
1   *teaspoon baking soda*
1   *teaspoon salt*
½   *teaspoon ground cinnamon*
¼   *teaspoon ground nutmeg*
⅛   *teaspoon ground cloves*
1   *tablespoon milled chia*
1   *(6 ounce) container vanilla low-fat yogurt (or coconut-based yogurt)*
¾   *cup mashed ripe banana (approximately 1½ bananas)*
¼   *teaspoon vanilla extract*

Optional: ½ cup chopped walnuts or pecans

1. Preheat the oven to 350°F.
2. Grease an 8 x 4-inch loaf pan with butter.
3. In a large mixing bowl, cream the butter and sugar. You can do this with a hand-held mixer or in a stand mixer. Beat at medium speed until fluffy and well blended.
4. Add the eggs, one at a time, beating well after each addition.
5. In a separate bowl, sift together the flour, baking soda, salt, cinnamon, nutmeg, cloves, and milled chia.
6. Alternating, add half of the flour mixture, all of the yogurt, then the remaining half of the flour mixture to sugar mixture, beating well after each addition.
7. Fold in the bananas, vanilla, and nuts, if using.
8. Pour the batter into the prepared loaf pan and place on middle rack in the oven.
9. Bake until a wooden toothpick inserted into the bread's center comes out clean, 50 to 60 minutes.
10. Cool for 10 minutes in the pan on a wire rack. Remove from the pan, slice and serve.

PUMPKIN BREAD

MAKES 6 TO 9 SERVINGS

Warm, spicy and luscious, this scrumptious bread is an autumn staple in many homes. What sets this version apart, however, is chia, which gives the finished product a moist texture and ultra-nutritious profile.

½ *stick butter, softened, plus more for greasing pan*

1 *teaspoon Stevia powder or equivalent other sugar substitute*

1 *large egg, lightly beaten (you can use 2 egg whites for less fat)*

½ *teaspoon orange extract or vanilla extract*

1 *cup canned pumpkin*

1¼ *cups all-purpose flour*

2 *teaspoons baking powder*

¾ *teaspoon baking soda*

½ *teaspoon salt*

1 *tablespoon milled chia*

1½ *teaspoons ground cinnamon*

¾ *teaspoon ground ginger*

¼ *teaspoon ground nutmeg*

Optional: ½ cup raisins

Optional: ⅓ cup chopped pecans

Optional: 3 tablespoons apricot jam or spreadable fruit (for glazed topping)

Optional: Pecan halves or chopped pecans, for garnish

1. Preheat the oven to 350 °F.

2. Grease an 8 x 4-inch loaf pan with butter.

3. With mixer, beat the butter and Stevia until blended.

4. Add in the egg, orange extract and pumpkin.

5. In a separate bowl, sift together the flour, baking powder, baking soda, salt, milled chia, cinnamon, ginger, and nutmeg.

6. Add the dry ingredients to the egg-pumpkin mixture a little at a time, beating until combined after each addition.

7. Add the raisins and chopped pecans, if using.

8. Spread the batter evenly into the greased loaf pan and place on middle rack in the oven. Bake until a toothpick inserted in the center of the bread comes out clean, 35-40 minutes.

9. Let bread sit 5 minutes after removing from the oven. Remove the bread from the pan and let it finish cooling on wire rack.

10. If using, heat the jam or spreadable fruit until melted; brush or spoon the glaze onto the loaf. Garnish with pecans, if using.

CAKE MIX MADE BETTER

Cake mixes are not the most nutritious kitchen helpers around, but when you're in a pinch, they make getting a dozen cupcakes made for your kids' school bake sale a snap. "Healthy-up" a store-bought cake mix with chia. Simply replace half of the recommended oil with chia gel (see page 77). If you're using pre-made frosting, you can also stir in a tablespoon of chia gel before spreading it onto the cake.

CHIA SNACK BARS
MAKES 9 TO 12 SERVINGS

This recipe yields a soft, granola-like snack bar, the type you often find in supermarket cereal aisles. This one, however, contains only the best ingredients: Coconut oil, chia, oats, nuts, dates, and chocolate. Yum!

¼ *cup virgin liquid coconut oil*
1 *tablespoon milled chia*
1 *cup chopped pitted Medjool dates or pitted prunes*
¼ *cup almond milk*
1 *teaspoon vanilla extract*
Optional: ½ teaspoon almond extract

1½ *cups rolled oats*
½ *cup whole wheat pastry flour*
⅓ *cup finely chopped nuts (use your favorite—one variety or a mix)*
¾ *teaspoon baking soda*
½ *teaspoon salt*
¼ *to ½ cup chopped dark chocolate or mini chocolate chips*

1. Preheat the oven to 350°F.
2. Using a food processor or a high-power blender (such as a Vitamix or Blendtec) combine the coconut oil, milled chia, dates, milk, vanilla extract, and almond extract. Pulse until a smooth paste has formed, scraping the sides down as needed.
3. In a large bowl, whisk together the oats, flour, nuts, baking soda, and salt, and combine thoroughly.
4. Add the chia mixture and the chopped chocolate to the flour mixture, mixing gently until just combined.
5. Spread the mixture onto a cookie sheet in a half-inch thick layer, creating a rectangle. Mixture will not reach the sides of the baking sheet.
6. Before putting the mixture into the oven, dip a knife into cold water and cut the mixture into 4 x 2-inch bars.
7. Bake on the middle rack until golden brown and set to the touch, 12 to 15 minutes.

LOW-FAT BAKING WITH CHIA

Fat gives baked goods the moist, tender texture so prized in baking. For anyone looking to cut the fat in their favorite muffin, bread, cookie, or cake recipe, chia can help. Chia gel (see recipe, page 77) can be used tablespoon for tablespoon as a replacement for the fat or oil in your favorite recipe: If your cake recipe calls for 8 tablespoons of butter, you can replace half of those with chia gel without affecting the results. Chia also gives baked goods moisture. If "Grandma's Favorite Chocolate Chip Cookies" recipe calls for 8 tablespoons of butter, use 4 tablespoons of butter and 4 tablespoons of chia gel without altering the taste or texture of your recipe.

When baking with chia—whether it's whole chia seeds, chia gel, or milled chia—you may find it takes longer for recipes to be done. Typically, recipes with chia need to be baked for about 5 percent longer than non-chia recipes. This means that a muffin recipe that takes 20 minutes to bake may require an extra minute (or two) when you add chia.

CHIA ON THE GO

Chia seed is fast. It's easy. It's good for you. But for those times when you don't want to eat anything, chia gel may be just what you need: Simply swirl a tablespoon of chia gel into a glass of room temperature water, drink and go. Voila! A deeply hydrating way to fill up and ward off hunger and cravings. A glass of this "chia water" is also great before meals to add bulk to the tummy, which in turn helps prevent overeating.

BREAKFAST FOODS

CHIA GEL

MAKES 1¼ CUPS

Many of the recipes in this book called for chia gel, a quick, easy staple you can whip up at home and store in your fridge. With a stash of chia gel at the ready, it's a cinch to increase the nutrient profile of your favorite foods. Add it to creamy foods, liquids, condiments, salad dressings, and even peanut butter and jelly. The gel doesn't affect flavors. What it does, however, is increase a food's vitamin and mineral levels, and add protein and omega fatty acids, while promoting weight loss by filling your stomach with fiber. Here is one way to make chia "gel."

1 cup cool water
1¾ tablespoons chia seeds

1. Pour the water into a sealable plastic or glass container. Slowly pour chia seeds into water while briskly mixing with wire whisk.
2. Wait 3 or 4 minutes then whisk again.
3. Let the mixture stand about 10 minutes before whisking again. Seal the container and store mixture in the refrigerator for up to two weeks to use as needed. Whisk before using. **Note:** Soaking in water will soften the chia seeds, but they will still be slightly crunchy.

CINNAMON-ORANGE PANCAKES

SERVES 4

Pancakes are the quintessential breakfast food, perfect for weekend mornings with the family. Not only are these eggless griddle cakes delicious and tremendously filling, they also pack a powerful wallop of nutrients and fiber. For an autumn treat, try them with a side of sautéed pears, apples, or quince.

¾ cup unbleached whole wheat pastry flour
1 cup oat flour
2 teaspoons baking powder
1 tablespoon brown sugar
1 teaspoon cinnamon
1 cup milk
¾ cup orange juice
¾ cup chia gel (see recipe, page 77)
Optional: 1 teaspoon grated orange zest
Vegetable oil, or cooking spray, as needed

1. In a large bowl, combine the dry ingredients. Wisk until thoroughly combined.
2. In another bowl, combine all the liquid ingredients, including chia gel and the orange zest, if using.
3. Pour the liquid ingredients into the dry ingredients and stir only until moistened.
4. Lightly grease a non-stick griddle with oil or cooking spray and preheat over medium heat. Ladle ½–¾ cup of the batter onto the grill, depending on the size you like.

5. Flip the pancakes when bubbles appear on the surface. Cook until the underside is golden brown.
6. Serve with Orange-Date Syrup (recipe follows) or your favorite pancake topping.

VEGAN-FRIENDLY PROTEIN

As we all know by now, chia offers a powerful wallop of protein. What you may not know is that chia is a *complete protein*, meaning that it contains all the amino acids your body needs to utilize this macronutrient. This is great news for anyone looking for a high quality protein source, but it is particularly helpful for vegans (vegetarians who eat nothing of animal origin, including dairy products, eggs, or honey). Because many plant sources have incomplete protein, many vegans find it difficult to get the protein they need without complicated food combining. Chia can solve this dilemma.

ORANGE DATE SYRUP

MAKES 2 CUPS

This luxurious syrup not only tastes decadent, it's actually packed with nutrition thanks to all the dates, orange juice, and chia. It's also fantastic stirred into plain yogurt, as a sauce for ham, or syrup for ice cream. Enjoy!

1   cup boiling water
1   cup pitted dates
¾   cup frozen orange juice
     concentrate, thawed
1   cup chia gel (see recipe,
     page 77)

1. Pour the boiling water over the dates in a bowl and let stand for 10 minutes. Mash them with a potato masher or the back of a fork.
2. Add the orange juice concentrate.
3. Pour the date-orange juice mixture into a blender and liquefy.
4. Remove from the blender and whisk in the chia gel, mixing until thoroughly combined.
5. Store in a jar in the refrigerator, shaking well before using.

CHIA FRENCH TOAST
SERVES 2 OR 3

Chia infuses what is traditionally a low-nutrient breakfast dish with fiber, vitamins, minerals, omegas, additional protein, and more. Give this a try and you'll find yourself feeling satiated and more energetic. Kids adore this!

2   large eggs
4   teaspoons chia gel (see recipe, page 77)
4   to 6 slices of whole wheat bread,
     preferably day old or slightly dry
     Vegetable oil or cooking spray, as needed

1. In a medium bowl, whisk the eggs until smooth.
2. Add the chia gel.
3. Dip the bread in the egg-chia mixture, coating both sides.
4. Heat a large skillet over medium heat and grease lightly with oil or cooking spray. Fry the soaked bread for 2 to 3 minutes until browned. Turn and repeat on the other side.
5. Serve with Chia Breakfast Syrup (see recipe, below) or the topping of your choice.

CHIA BREAKFAST SYRUP
MAKES ½ CUP

Your favorite breakfast syrup just got healthier! This easy recipe is great for pancakes, waffles, French toast—and even as an ice cream topper.

2   teaspoons chia gel (see recipe, page 77)
½   cup maple or fruit syrup. (This keeps
     indefinitely in the refrigerator in a tightly
     closed jar.)

1. In a large bowl, whisk the chia gel and syrup until smooth.
2. Store in a tightly closed jar for up to two weeks in the refrigerator.

CHIA SPREAD

You can make your own sweet nut butter spread that's perfect for quick sand-wiches, graham-cracker treats, or topping apple slices. Here's how: combine ½ cup nut butter of your choice (almond, cashew, sunflower, sesame seed, peanut) and ¼ cup of your favorite syrup (maple, fruit, Chia Breakfast Syrup) with 1 tablespoon chia seeds. Mix thoroughly. This keeps in the refrigerator in a tightly closed jar for two weeks.

SCRAMBLED CHIA EGGS

SERVES 1 TO 2

If you typically have two eggs for breakfast, you may find yourself eating less with this recipe. That's because the chia expands in your stomach, creating a pleasant sensation of full-ness while delivering an infusion of nutrients.

2 *large eggs*
1 *teaspoon chia gel (see recipe, page 77)*
   Vegetable oil or cooking spray, as needed

1. In a medium bowl, whisk the eggs until smooth.
2. Add chia gel and whisk until combined.
3. Heat a frying pan over medium-low heat and grease lightly with vegetable oil or cooking spray. Pour in the eggs and cook, stirring gently, until eggs are scrambled.

CHIA FRITTATA

SERVES 2

This easy recipe is a terrific way to finish last night's leftover cooked veggies. Use what-ever you have on hand—this delicious recipe is infinitely flexible. Serve it up with a green salad for a fast, nutrient-rich supper.

3 *large eggs*
1 *teaspoon chia gel (see recipe, page 77)*
¼ to ½ *cup chopped cooked veggies*
   Vegetable oil, as needed

1. In a medium bowl, whisk the eggs until smooth.
2. Add the chia gel and whisk until combined.
3. Add the vegetables and stir until combined.
4. Heat a frying pan over medium heat and grease lightly with oil. Pour in the egg mix-ture and cook, without stirring, until eggs are set completely through.
5. Allow to cool in the pan slightly before sliding the frittata onto a cutting board. Cut into wedges to serve.

CHIA EGG TOPPERS

If you love your eggs with ketchup, salsa, or chili sauce, there's yet another way to work chia into your diet. Simply mix ½ cup of your favorite condiment with 1 tablespoon chia. Store it in the refrigerator in a tightly closed jar for up to two weeks.

RAW VANILLA COCONUT "YOGURT"

SERVES 1 OR 2

This luscious yogurt is ideal for those who don't eat dairy. Smooth and creamy, it's the creation of Jackie Rafter. Easy and quick to prepare, this recipe makes a delicious, filling breakfast all on its own or as an accompaniment to your favorite cold cereal.

1 to 2 tablespoons chia seeds
1 cup dried (desiccated) coconut
1 cup fresh filtered water or coconut water
*   (more or less to your preference)*
1 tablespoon raw agave, maple syrup, honey,
*   or a shake of Stevia*
1 teaspoon vanilla extract
1 teaspoon hazelnut or almond extract
*   (optional)*
*   Pinch of sea salt*
Optional topping: Fresh fruits or berries and
*   honey or raw agave syrup*

1. Place all the ingredients, except optional fruit topping, in a blender or food processor. Process until the yogurt is smooth and creamy.

CHIA BREAKFAST SANDWICH

If you or your kids find it difficult to find time for a sit-down breakfast, here's an easy grab-and-go option called the Chia-Nut Butter Sandwich. Take two pieces of prepared French toast or bread of your choice (whole wheat, non-gluten, rye, etc.). Spread one slice with almond butter (or sunflower seed butter, tahini, peanut butter, or cashew butter). Sprinkle two teaspoons of chia seeds over the nut butter. Spread the remaining slice with honey, maple syrup, agave, or a low-sugar jelly and place on top of the nut butter-chia slice. Delicious and fast.

2. Add more water or coconut if necessary to make more of a "yogurt" consistency.

3. Serve in a bowl and top with fresh fruits and/or berries. Decorate with a swirl of honey or raw agave syrup and enjoy! Store leftover yogurt in the refrigerator and simply add more water if a creamier texture is desired later on.

CHIA-OAT PORRIDGE

SERVES 2

Oatmeal and chia are a natural pairing, creating a wholesome, nourishing, stay-with-you breakfast that benefits the heart while helping dieters lose weight. Garnish this old-fashioned porridge with dried fruit, fresh fruit, honey, maple syrup, or anything else that strikes your fancy.

1¾ cup water
¾ cup old fashioned rolled oats (sometimes called 5-minute oats)
Dash salt
1 tablespoon chia seeds
Optional: 1 teaspoon butter or coconut oil

1. Place the water in small pot over medium high heat.

2. When the water comes to a rolling boil, add the oats, salt, and butter or coconut oil, if using. Stir once and reduce the heat to low.

3. After five minutes, remove from the heat. Stir in the chia seeds and serve immediately.

FAST CHIA BREAKFASTS

Chia is so easy to use that there is no need to whip up a special recipe to enjoy it. Simply add it to your current favorite breakfast foods. Here are some ideas:

- Sprinkle up to 1 tablespoon of chia, depending on your taste, over cold cereal or a bowl of oatmeal.
- Layer fruit, yogurt, and a sprinkle of chia seeds into a glass for a breakfast parfait.
- Add chia to your favorite pancake or waffle recipe (or mix).
- Sprinkle chia onto waffles before cooking or onto pancakes before turning.
- Add a dusting of chia seeds to an omelet before turning it out of the pan.
- Spoon scrambled eggs, salsa, black beans, and chia seeds into a tortilla before rolling to make a healthy breakfast wrap.

CHIA-QUINOA PORRIDGE

SERVES TWO

Superfood meets superfood in this powerful porridge of champions. Pronounced *keen-wah*, quinoa is a small seed that is treasured in the Andes for its high amino acid profile, protein, and high levels of magnesium and iron. When teamed up with chia, the two create one of the most nutrient-dense breakfasts around.

1½ cup water or milk (dairy, rice, almond, hemp, coconut, etc.)
1 cup quinoa, quickly rinsed in a colander
Dash salt
1 tablespoon chia seeds
Optional: 1 teaspoon butter or coconut oil

1. Place the water or milk in a small pot over medium-high heat.

2. When the water comes to a rolling boil, add the quinoa, salt, and butter or coconut oil, if using. Stir once, cover, and reduce the heat to lowest setting.
3. Check after 10 minutes. If the grain is soft, remove from the heat, stir in the chia seeds and serve immediately.

CHIANOLA

MAKES 12 CUPS

Granola is so fun and easy to make that you have no excuse not to give it a try. Think of this recipe as a canvas for your creativity. You can swap pumpkin seeds or hazelnuts for the almonds, almond extract for the vanilla, and so on. You'll notice this version is much leaner than commercially available granolas—it's also much lower in sugar. The addition of chia adds a high impact boost of nutrients, as well as filling fiber.

4   cups quick-cooking oats
½   cup oat bran
½   cup unsweetened dried (dessicated) coconut
¼ to ⅓ cup chopped almonds
    Dash salt
1 to 2 tablespoons chia seeds
¼   cup coconut milk
¼   cup virgin coconut oil
⅓   cup maple syrup
¼   cup apple juice
Optional: ½ teaspoon vanilla extract
Optional: ¼ cup chopped dried fruit

1. Preheat oven to 350°F.
2. In a large bowl, combine the dry ingredients until well blended.
3. In a small pot over medium heat, bring the coconut milk, coconut oil, maple syrup, and apple juice to a boil and cook for two minutes.
4. Remove from the heat and stir in the vanilla extract, if using. Pour the mixture into the dry ingredients, stirring thoroughly to coat.
5. Divide the mixture between two baking sheets and bake until granola is golden and fragrant, about 7 or 8 minutes.
6. Cool the granola on the pans. Stir in the dried fruit, if using.
7. Store the granola in an airtight container in a cool, dry spot.

MORE CALCIUM

Dairy products are not the only way to give your body the calcium it needs. Chia seeds are rich in this important bone-building mineral. Ounce for ounce, chia has five times more calcium than the same amount of cow's milk. Chia also contains boron, a trace element that helps transfer calcium into the bones.

AUSSIE-STYLE BROILED TOMATOES WITH CHIA
SERVES TWO

A broiled tomato half—often with a scattering of scrumptious browned crumbs—is a breakfast staple down under, served as part of a traditional Aussie breakfast of canned apricots and beans on toast. Don't have any beans in your pantry? No worries—this savory side dish is wonderful with anything, even by itself as a snack.

1   beefsteak tomato
2   tablespoons bread crumbs
1   teaspoon olive oil or melted butter
1   teaspoon chia seeds
    Dash salt and pepper

1. Preheat the broiler.
2. Slice the tomato in half cross-wise, through the middle. Place the tomato halves on a broiler-proof pan.

ACID TAMER

Tomatoes contain citric and malic acids, making them difficult for some people to digest comfortably. If you experience a sour stomach, heartburn, or other digestive upsets after eating tomatoes, a sprinkle of chia might help. How it works: Chia absorbs the stomach-sizzling acids in tart foods in the same way it absorbs water, which could be just the right way to help you enjoy a tomato-rich, acidic food, without the usual discomfort.

3. In a small bowl, combine the breadcrumbs, oil or butter, salt, and pepper. Spoon the mixture onto each tomato half.

4. Place the tomato halves under the broiler until the topping is golden and the tomato slightly softened. Remove from the oven and sprinkle the chia seeds over the tomatoes before serving.

LUNCH

FAST SOUP
SERVES ONE OR TWO

This is a "treatment" for canned soup more than it is a recipe, and it makes a fast, low-fat lunch—great to eat when you're hungry for something quick and nutritious.

1   12-ounce can soup or chili of your choice (no-additive brands such as Amy's, Health Valley, and Muir Glen are preferable)
1 or 2 tablespoons chia gel (see recipe, page 77)

1. Heat the soup in a small pot over medium-low heat, or according to directions.

2. Remove from the heat and swirl in chia gel.

SOUPED-UP SOUPS

Before you add chia gel, chia seeds, or milled chia to soups, stews, and chili, turn off the heat and wait a few moments for the liquid to cool a little bit before swirling in the chia. This way, you'll get the full complement of chia's many nutrients.

LIMA BEAN WINTER SOUP

MAKES 6 TO 8 SERVINGS

Named after the capitol of Peru, lima beans are soft, buttery, and full of minerals, protein, and cholesterol-lowering fiber. Feel free to try the recipe with white navy beans or cannellini beans.

2 *cups dried lima beans, soaked overnight*
8 *cups chicken or vegetable broth, plus more as needed*
¼ *cup extra-virgin olive oil*
1 *large onion, finely chopped*
2 *garlic cloves, minced*
2 *carrots, finely chopped*
⅛ *teaspoon cayenne pepper*
1 *teaspoon dried parsley*
½ *red bell pepper, chopped*
½ *green bell pepper, chopped*
½ *cup chia gel (see recipe, page 77)*
   Salt to taste

1. Place the beans and broth in a stockpot or large saucepan over medium-high heat. Boil for 10 minutes.
2. Lower the heat and simmer until the beans are tender, about 30 minutes. Add more broth or water as needed.
3. Add the olive oil to a frying pan over medium heat and sauté the onions, garlic, carrots, cayenne, and dried parsley until the vegetables are tender, about 3 minutes.
4. Add the sautéed mixture to lima beans. Stir to combine.

5. Add the red and green peppers and chia gel to the pot and simmer the soup for 20 minutes to allow the flavors to meld.

CREAMY MUSHROOM-CASHEW SOUP

MAKES 4 TO 6 SERVINGS

Cashew milk is a vegan mainstay, prized for its creamy, rich, comforting taste. Here, cashew milk combines with mushrooms and chia to create a delectable soup. Add a green salad and a bit of protein and you have yourself a delicious, well-rounded meal!

1 *cup raw cashews, washed thoroughly in hot water*
5½ *cups chicken or vegetable broth or water*
1½ *tablespoons dry chia seeds*
1½ *tablespoons butter*
1 *pound sliced mushrooms, mixed varieties if possible*
2 *tablespoons extra-virgin olive oil*
1½ *medium yellow or sweet onions (such as Maui, Vidalia, or Walla Walla), diced*
2 *celery stalks, with leaves, diced*
2 *cloves garlic, chopped*
1 *teaspoon cold-pressed toasted sesame oil*
1 *teaspoon tamari*
1½ *teaspoons dried basil*
½ *teaspoon salt, or to taste*
⅛ *teaspoon cayenne pepper, or to taste*
Optional: 1 medium tomato, seeded and chopped, as garnish

1. In a food processor or high-power blender (such as Vitamix or Blendtec), process the cashews with the broth or water to make cashew milk.

2. Stir the chia seeds into the cashew milk and let stand for 15 minutes.

3. Melt the butter in a sauté pan over medium heat. Add half of the mushrooms and sauté for about 4 minutes.

4. Add the sautéed mushrooms to the food processor or blender with the cashew milk-chia mixture and blend until smooth.

5. Heat the olive oil in a large pot over medium heat and sauté the onions, celery and garlic until soft.

6. Stir in the sesame oil and tamari, and remaining mushrooms. Sauté until the mushrooms are just soft.

7. Add the pureed cashew-mushroom mixture to the pot and simmer the soup for 15 minutes.

8. Add the basil, salt, and cayenne pepper to taste.

9. Stir in the chopped tomato immediately before serving.

CASHEW TRIVIA

Cashews are the darlings of the snack world because they are lower in fat than other nuts, higher in protein, and addictively delicious. You know you love them, but did you know this about them?:

- Cashews are native to the coastal regions of northeastern Brazil.
- The cashew nut is actually the kidney-shaped seed that sits at the bottom of the cashew apple, a delicacy in Brazil and the Caribbean, where the fruit grows prolifically.
- Cashews are always sold shelled. Why? Because the interior of the cashew shell contains a caustic resin known as cashew balm, which is carefully removed before nuts are packaged for human consumption. This resin is used to make insecticides and varnishes.
- Cashew's scientific name is *Anacardium occidentale*.
- Cashews belong to the same family as the pistachio and mango.
- In the 16th century, Portuguese explorers took cashew trees from Brazil and introduced them to other tropical countries, including India and Africa.
- Currently, the leading commercial providers of cashews are Brazil, Mozambique, Tanzania, and Nigeria.
- Cashew wood is a precious, much-prized resource in Brazil.

MULLIGATAWNY CHIA SOUP
SERVES 6

This is one of those delicious recipes that everyone loves. It's also supremely versatile. Try adding a bit of leftover rice or some chopped chicken or lamb, and garnish with a flourish of nuts. Have fun playing with this one!

5   cups vegetable or chicken stock, plus
      more as needed (you can substitute one
      cup coconut milk for one cup of broth)
1   cup red lentils
½   teaspoon turmeric
Optional: 1 teaspoon Madras curry powder
1   medium potato, diced
5   cloves garlic, minced
1¼ inch piece fresh ginger root, peeled and
      finely grated
¼   teaspoon cayenne
1   teaspoon ground coriander
1   tablespoon lemon juice
3   tablespoons liquid virgin coconut oil
1½ cups chia gel (see recipe, page 77)
      Salt and black pepper to taste

1. In a large pot over medium heat, combine the broth, lentils, turmeric, curry powder (if using), and potato. Simmer until the lentils and potatoes are soft, 10 to 15 minutes. Add additional broth, water, or coconut milk as needed.
2. Add the garlic, ginger, cayenne, coriander, lemon juice, coconut oil, and chia gel and simmer for 10 minutes to meld flavors.
3. Add salt and black pepper as needed.

MULLIGA-WHAT?

The word mulligatawny is an anglicized version of a Tamil word meaning "pepper broth." This spicy soup became a favorite of Britains during the colonization of India in the late 18th century. As the dish migrated back to England and through the British Commonwealth, it began to mutate. Some versions omitted the original curry, others left out the coconut milk, while some recipes added cilantro, used chicken broth, instead of the original mutton broth, and even included chopped apples or nuts. In other words, this is a soup to be played with. Feel free to add or subtract to it at will!

POWER WRAP
MAKES 1

Wraps are fun to make and easy to eat. They are also supremely versatile. This protein-packed version can be updated and customized any way you like.

2   tablespoons hummus, plain or flavored
1   tablespoon chia gel (see recipe, page 77)
1   large tortilla or wrap of choice (we like
      whole grain or gluten-free versions)
Optional: A pinch of black pepper or a few
      dashes of hot sauce

1   tablespoon sunflower seeds
¼   cup shredded carrots
2   Romaine or other lettuce leaves
¼ to ½ of an avocado, thinly sliced lengthwise

1. In a small bowl, whisk together the hummus, chia gel, and pepper or hot sauce, if using.

2. Lay the wrap on a flat surface. Spread the hummus-chia mixture over the surface of the wrap, stopping about a half-inch before reaching the wrap's edges.

3. Sprinkle sunflower seeds over the hummus, leaving a two-inch margin at the bottom of the wrap. This will make rolling easier and cleaner.

4. Layer on the shredded carrots, lettuce, and avocado slices, being careful to leave a two-inch margin at the bottom of the wrap.

5. Starting at the top, roll the wrap into a tube. Squeeze the rolled wrap gently to seal.

EASY ADDITION

Almost any condiment, dip, or spread can be enhanced with the addition of chia gel (see recipe, page 77). Feel free to experiment, but if you'd like some guidance, start here:

- **Nut butter:** Add up to 1 tablespoon chia gel for every tablespoon nut butter.
- **Jam or jelly:** Add 1 teaspoon chia gel for every tablespoon jam or jelly.
- **Maple syrup or honey:** Add 1 teaspoon chia gel for every tablespoon of syrup.
- **Mayonnaise:** Add up to 1 tablespoon chia gel for every tablespoon mayo.
- **Mustard:** Add up to 1 tablespoon chia gel for every tablespoon mustard.
- **Ketchup and cocktail sauce:** Add 1 teaspoon chia gel for every tablespoon ketchup or cocktail sauce.
- **Barbecue sauce:** Add 1 teaspoon chia gel for every tablespoon barbecue sauce.
- **Guacamole:** Add ½ tablespoon chia gel for every tablespoon of guacamole.
- **Hummus and other bean dips:** Add 1 tablespoon chia gel for every tablespoon hummus.
- **Salsa:** Add 1 teaspoon chia gel for every tablespoon salsa.
- **Salad dressing:** Add 1 tablespoon chia gel for every tablespoon salad dressing.
- **Sour cream:** Add 1 tablespoon chia for every tablespoon sour cream.

CHIA HUMMUS

Looking for a quick, healthy dip for veggie sticks, rice crackers, tortilla chips, and other dippers? Place a small garlic clove, ½ cup hummus, ¼ cup salsa, and 2 tablespoons chia gel (see recipe, page 77) into a food processor. Pulse until the mixture forms a smooth paste. Use it as a dip or a great sandwich spread.

CHIA SALAD SANDWICH

MAKES ENOUGH FOR 1 OR 2 SANDWICHES

Chicken and turkey salad, egg and tuna salad—most people love these protein-rich sandwich fillings. In this version, you get to pick your favorite protein, then dress it up with high-mileage veggies, seasonings, and chia.

3 *tablespoons low fat mayonnaise or plain yogurt*
1 *tablespoon chia gel (see recipe, page 77)*
1 *tablespoon mustard (yellow, Dijon, spicy brown, or any type you enjoy)*
1 *6-ounce can tuna, salmon, or 1 cup chopped chicken, turkey, hardboiled eggs, ham, tofu, tempeh, or seitan*
¼ *cup shredded or minced carrots*
¼ *cup chopped red onion*
¼ *cup chopped celery*
¼ *cup chopped red bell pepper (fresh or jarred)*
1 *tablespoon chopped fresh parsley, cilantro, or dill*

Bread slices, wrap, or crackers of your choice
Optional: Romaine lettuce for garnish

1. In a large bowl, mix the mayonnaise, chia gel, and mustard, whisking until smooth.
2. Add the tuna or protein of choice, carrots, onion, celery, red pepper, and herb of choice, mixing until combined.
3. Spoon onto the bread or wrap, topping with lettuce. Or, use to top crackers.

TUNA WITHOUT THE MERCURY?

Tuna and other large, oily sea fish are typically high in mercury. This is because these fish spend years absorbing mercury and other heavy metals that enter the oceans as pollution. Most canned tuna has at least 13 percent more mercury than the 0.5 ppm maximum declared safe by the USDA. You can lower your exposure to mercury and other heavy metals by using "light" tuna instead of "white" tuna.

CURRIED POTATO SALAD

MAKES 8 SERVINGS

Don't like mayo? Don't eat eggs? You'll love this flavorful vegan salad. Of course if you have to have your mayo, go ahead and swap it for the tofu and oil.

1   carton soft tofu
¼   cup extra-virgin olive oil
¼   cup chia gel (see recipe, page 77)
1   teaspoon Dijon mustard
1½ teaspoons mild curry powder
½   teaspoon cumin powder
½   teaspoon cayenne pepper
12 red potatoes, boiled, cooled, and cut into
    large cubes
1   red onion, chopped
½   green bell pepper, chopped
½   red bell pepper, chopped
1   Serrano chili pepper, minced
½   bunch flat leaf parsley, minced
1   cup celery, finely chopped
    Salt to taste

1. In a food processor or high-speed blender (such as Vitamix or BlendTex) process the tofu and olive oil until smooth.
2. Add the chia gel, mustard, curry powder, cumin, and cayenne, processing until smooth.
3. In a large bowl, gently combine the potatoes, onion, peppers, parsley, and celery.
4. Add dressing to potatoes, combining gently to coat, and season with salt.
5. Serve immediately or refrigerate until ready to serve.

DOES CURRY PROMOTE WEIGHT LOSS?

Depending upon whom you ask, *curry* comes from the Tamil word *kari*, which means sauce, or, it refers to curry leaves (also known as sweet neem leaves), one of the ingredients in curry powder.

Typically a mixture of turmeric, cumin, cinnamon, fennel, ginger, chili peppers, and black pepper, curry powder is touted as a weight loss aid by some weight loss gurus. Most likely it's the turmeric at work. This bright yellow spice helps lower LDL ("bad") cholesterol. But other ingredients may help pare down pounds, as well: A Dutch study found that turmeric and its "curry mates," cumin, chili, black pepper, and ginger all help to rev up the metabolism, speeding the amount of calories the body burns.

MEXICAN GRAIN PILAF
SERVES 2 TO 4

Think of this fun recipe as a guide—it was made to be customized. You can use millet, quinoa, barley, brown rice—or any cooked grain—as the base. Then mix in vegetables, pumpkin seeds, beans, and chia. This is a great lunchbox dish. If you want to really speed up prep time, buy pre-cooked frozen grain in the freezer section of your favorite grocer or health food store, then thaw and rinse what you need in hot water before serving.

1 to 2 tablespoons chia gel (see recipe, page 77)
1   tablespoon extra-virgin olive oil
1   teaspoon lime juice
½ teaspoon salt
Optional: A few shakes of Tabasco or other
    hot sauce
2   cups cooked brown rice, millet, quinoa,
    barley faro or other grain
½ cup cooked corn
½ cup cooked black beans
¼ cup chopped red onion
¼ cup chopped red bell pepper
¼ cup pepitas (green, hull-less pumpkin seeds)
½ to 1 tablespoons chopped cilantro

1. In a large bowl, whisk together the chia gel, olive oil, lime juice, salt, and hot sauce, if using.
2. Add the grain, corn, beans, onions, peppers, pepitas, and cilantro, stirring gently yet thoroughly to coat.

PUMPKIN POWER

Hull-less green pumpkin seeds—called pepitas in Spanish—are the perfect accompaniment to chia. High in vitamin E, niacin, iron, magnesium, manganese, and zinc, as well as tryptophan and oleic acid (which helps lower "bad" LDL cholesterol and raise "good" HDL cholesterol), these addictive kernels are delicious toasted in a dry skillet until they pop.

CHIA RICE SALAD
MAKES 6 SERVINGS

Rice salads are a terrific picnic food. They tuck into lunch boxes easily and make the perfect side dish, too. This fun version features classic Mediterranean flavors. Feel free to play with different veggies and herbs if you'd like.

½ cup chia gel (see recipe, page 77)
2   tablespoons extra-virgin olive oil
2   tablespoons lemon juice
1 to 2 cloves of garlic, minced
½ teaspoon salt
1   teaspoon fresh rosemary or oregano leaves,
    minced
⅛ teaspoon cayenne pepper
3   cups cooked brown rice (long grain, basmati,
    or short grain)
1   small zucchini, julienned
1   medium tomato, seeded and chopped
Optional: 2 tablespoons grated Parmesan cheese

1. In a small bowl, combine the chia gel, oil, lemon, garlic, salt, herbs, and cayenne. Whisk until well-blended. (You can also put ingredients into a tightly closed jar and shake vigorously to mix.)
2. In a large bowl, combine the rice, vegetables, and Parmesan cheese, if using.
3. Pour the dressing over the rice mixture, combining gently and thoroughly.

MOROCCAN CARROT SALAD

MAKES 4 TO 6 SERVINGS

Carrot salad is a classic side dish—fresh, cleansing, and satisfying. This version is made heartier (and healthier) with the addition of chia.

¼ cup chia gel (see recipe, page 77)
2 tablespoons extra-virgin olive oil
½ tablespoon lemon juice
3 cloves garlic, minced
1 teaspoon cumin
¼ teaspoon white or black pepper
 (or ⅛ teaspoon cayenne pepper)

8 carrots, grated (or use food processor with grating attachment)
Salt, to taste
Crushed red pepper to taste
Optional: White sesame seeds for garnish

1. In a large bowl, whisk together the chia gel, olive oil, lemon juice, garlic, cumin, and pepper.
2. Add the shredded carrots and gently mix to combine and evenly coat the carrots.
3. Season with salt and crushed red pepper. Garnish with white sesame seeds, if using.

CARROT LORE

Most of us grew up eating carrots—crunching raw carrot sticks or baby carrots after school, roasted carrots for dinner, shredded carrots in salad, and even downing carrot juice. Here are a few fun facts about this beloved veggie:

- Carrots are related to parsley, parsnips, anise, caraway, cumin, and dill.
- Carrots and their cousins are members of the *umbrelliferae* plant family, so called for the umbrella-like leaves and flower-clusters they produce.
- In the United States, carrot greens are not eaten, but in France and other European countries the leaves are minced into salads and soups, where their fresh, slightly bitter taste is greatly prized.
- Before the 15th century, orange carrots were nowhere to be seen; only purple, yellow, red, and white carrots were cultivated. These old varieties are making a comeback in green markets and farm stands across the country.
- One-third of all carrots consumed in the world are grown in China. Russia is the second largest producer, with the U.S. coming in third.
- California grows 80 percent of America's carrot crop, followed closely by Michigan, then Texas, illustrating that carrots have a very wide growth habitat.
- The average adult in the U.S. consumes 12 pounds of carrots a year.

CHIA FRUIT SALAD

MAKES 6 SERVINGS

Consider this recipe as a mere suggestion. Don't have apples? Use pears. Peaches aren't in season? Use strawberries. Be flexible, have fun, and enjoy.

3   *peaches, pitted and diced*
2   *apples, cored and diced*
2   *cups seedless grapes*
2   *cups fresh pineapple, diced*
2   *bananas, diced*
    Juice of ½ large lemon
2   *cups Chia Sunshine Sauce (see below)*

1. Gently combine peaches, apples, grapes, pineapple, bananas, and lemon juice in a large bowl.
2. Drizzle with Chia Sunshine Sauce, stirring gently just to coat.

CHIA SUNSHINE SAUCE

MAKES ABOUT 2 CUPS

This light, fruity sauce is fantastic on fruit salad or mesclun, or drizzled over Greek yogurt. It can also be used as a dessert sauce or dip for apple and pear slices. If you'd like tangier, slightly more acidic flavor, add a squirt of lemon or lime juice.

1   *large mango, peeled and chopped, or 1 cup*
    frozen mango, thawed

2   *bananas*
½   *cup chia gel (see recipe, page 77)*
2   *tablespoons maple syrup*

1. Process all the ingredients in a food processor or high-power blender (such as a Vitamix or Blendtec) until smooth and creamy.

ZIPPY SALAD DRESSING

MAKES 2 CUPS

You know that special sauce that a certain fast food chain puts on its burgers? Well, this is the healthy version. It's great with burgers of all kinds, and is delicious on green salads and potato salads. You can even drizzle it on chicken or fish.

1   *cup low-fat or regular mayonnaise*
½   *cup tomato juice*
½   *cup chia gel (see recipe, page 77)*
1   *teaspoon minced parsley*
1   *teaspoon minced chives*
¼   *teaspoon garlic salt*
¼   *teaspoon celery salt*

1. In a medium bowl, whisk all the ingredients together until smooth.
2. Use on garden salads or to dress pasta, grain, or potato salads.
3. Store tightly covered in the refrigerator for up to a week.

SNACKS

HIGH POWER CHIA CHIPS
AS MANY AS YOU WANT TO MAKE

This recipe may be worth the price of this book! Chia Chips are easy to make, easy to eat, and densely packed with an outrageous amount of protein, fiber, and nutrients. Bet you can't eat just one!

Cooking spray, or virgin coconut oil, for greasing pan
Chia gel, the amount of your choice (see recipe, page 77)
Optional: Sea salt, herb seasoning, or other flavoring

1. Preheat oven to 170°F.
2. Spray a clean baking sheet with a light coat of cooking spray or a thin layer of virgin coconut oil.
3. For each chip, spoon a teaspoon-sized amount of the chia gel onto the prepared cookie sheet, three inches apart. Transfer the pan to the oven.
4. Leave the pan in oven for 12 hours or overnight. The finished chips will resemble potato chips.
5. Optional: Sprinkle with salt and/or seasoning of your choice before serving.

PROTEIN BITES
MAKES 8 TO 10 BALLS

This powerful treat is just sweet enough to satisfy your cravings, but not so sweet that it'll send you on a roller coaster ride of sugar highs and lows. Concentrated with protein, fiber, and B-complex vitamins, a Protein Bite is the perfect snack to have, right before heading out for a run or to the gym. Kids love these, too.

1 cup nut butter (almond, cashew, sunflowerseed, sesame paste, etc.)

¼ cup pitted dates

¼ cup natural cacao powder (can use regular unsweetened cocoa or carob powder if you'd like)

3 tablespoons chia seeds

1 tablespoon virgin coconut oil

1 teaspoon cinnamon

Pinch of salt

Optional 1 tablespoon spirulina

Optional coating: 2 tablespoons chia seeds, chopped nuts, desiccated coconut, cacao nibs, chopped goji berries, etc.

MAKE YOUR OWN NUT BUTTER

If you have a food processor or a high-power blender, such as a Vitamix or Blendtec, making your own nut butter is a cinch! Simply add any quantity of raw or roasted nuts or seeds (you can even use a blend) to the machine and process until smooth. This may take up to 15 minutes, depending on the ingredients you use and your machine. Some people like to add a bit of salt or sweetener (maple syrup or honey are particularly good) or a teaspoon or more of virgin coconut oil to give the nut butter a silkier texture. Store nut butter in the refrigerator.

---

1. Place all the ingredients in a food processor or high-power blender (such as a Vitamix or Blendtec) and pulse until the mixture is smooth. Do not over-process—you do not want to liquefy the mixture.

2. Form the mixture into balls the size of a walnut. If desired, roll in chia seed, chopped nuts, desiccated coconut, cacao nibs, or anything else that appeals to you.

3. Store in the freezer.

ALEGRIA

MAKES ABOUT 6 SERVINGS

The word *alegria* means happiness in Spanish. It's also the name of an ancient popped amaranth candy popular in Mexico and Central America.

6 tablespoons amaranth

¼ cup chia seeds

¼ cup virgin coconut oil, *plus more for greasing pan*

¼ cup honey

¼ cup molasses

½ teaspoon vanilla extract

1. Pop the amaranth, one tablespoon at a time, into a very hot, dry skillet, until all the grains have popped. Transfer the popped grains to a shallow bowl before adding the next tablespoon to the skillet.

2. Toast the chia seed in the same pan, mixing the toasted chia with the popped amaranth.

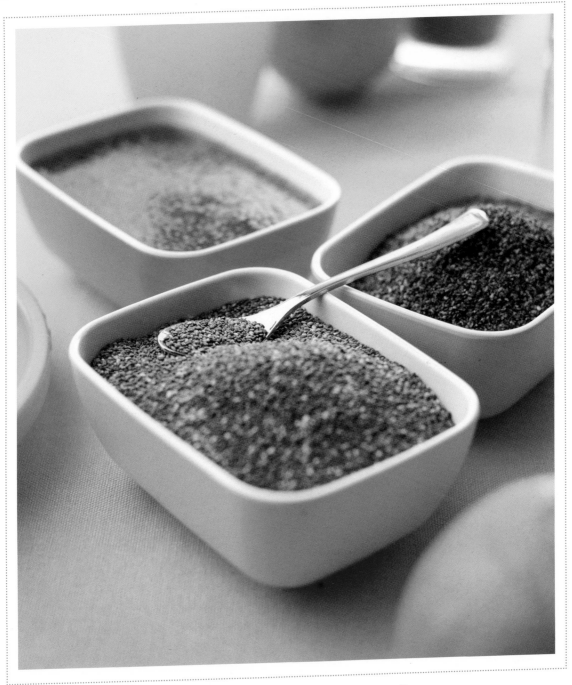

Chia seeds (foreground); milled chia (right); chia gel (background)

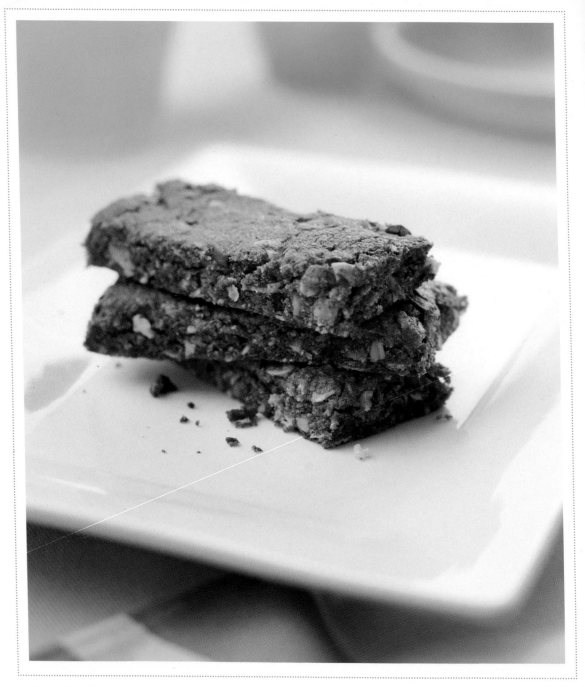

Chia Snack Bars, page 76

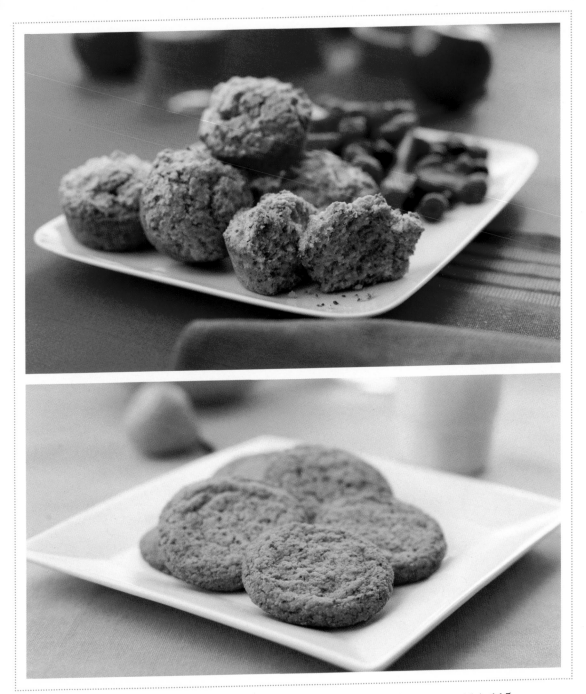

Top: Chia Seed Muffins, page 71; *Bottom:* Nut Butter Chia Cookies, pages 114–115

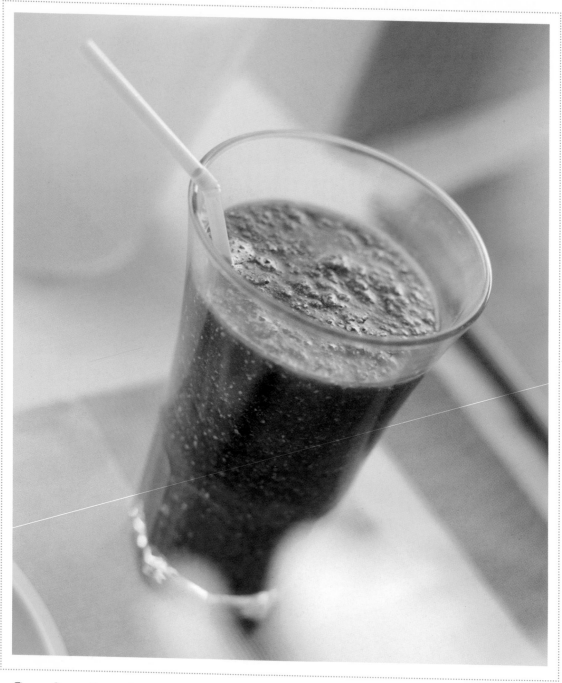

Green Super Smoothie, page 66

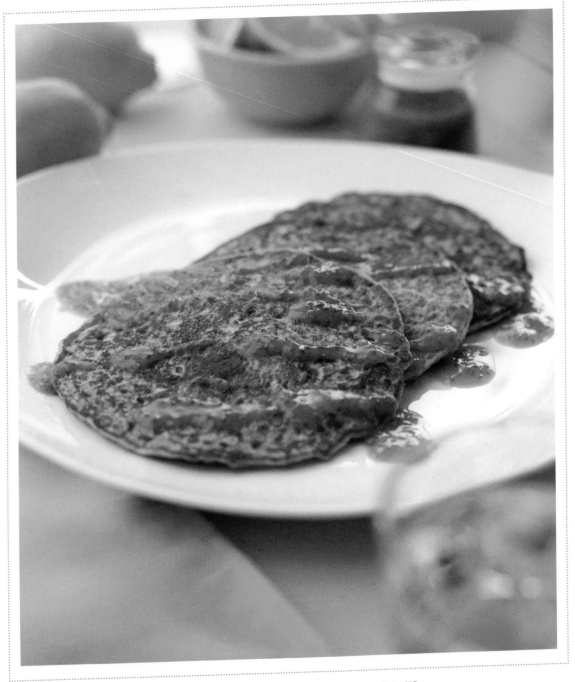

Cinnamon-Orange Pancakes with Orange Date Syrup, pages 78–79

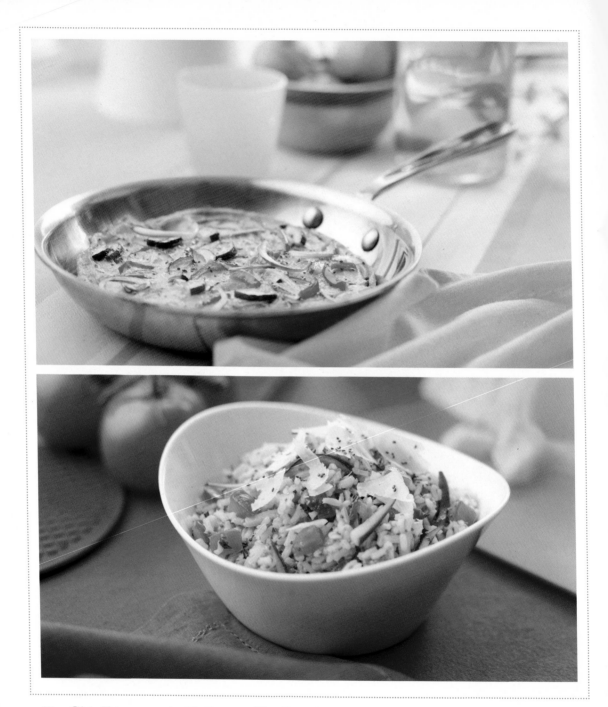

Top: Chia Frittata, page 80; *Bottom:* Chia Rice Salad, page 92

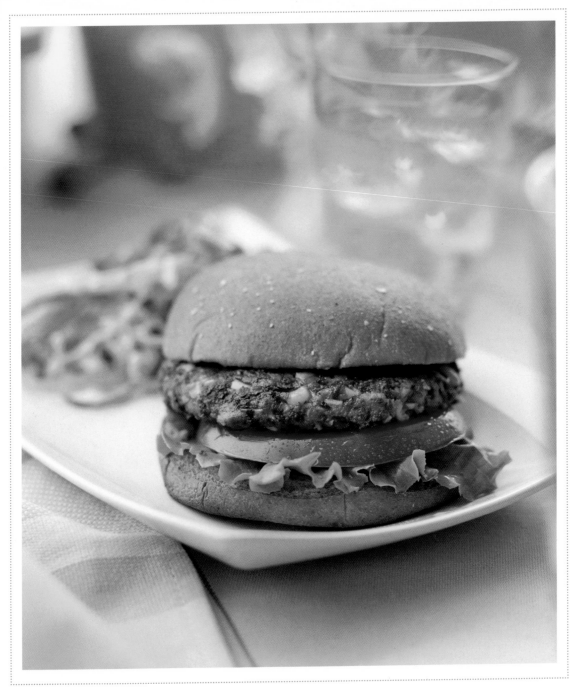

Chia Chipotle Bean Burger, page 107

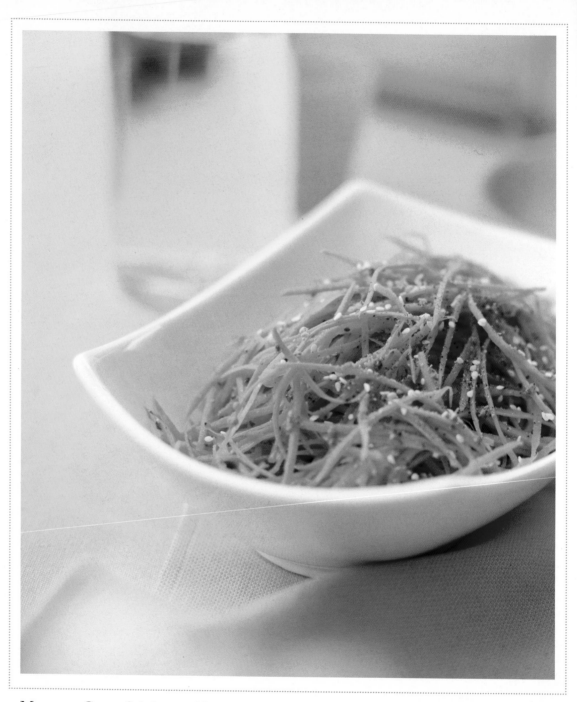

Moroccan Carrot Salad, page 93

3. Lightly coat a baking sheet with coconut oil.

4. In a heavy pot with a lid, combine the coconut oil, honey, molasses, and vanilla over medium-high heat. Cook until boiling, and then reduce heat to medium. Cook, stirring constantly, until the mixture turns dark amber and thickens, about 10 minutes.

5. Remove the mixture from heat and stir in the amaranth and chia, mixing well.

6. Spoon the mixture onto the prepared pan, spreading evenly into a thin layer.

7. Allow the mixture to cool and then cut into bars.

CHIA PÂTÉ

MAKES 2 CUPS

This elegant pâté is ideal for your next holiday meal or dinner party. Spread it on crackers or good bread—or use it as a dip for veggie sticks or a spread to replace mayo on sandwiches.

1   *cup raw cashews, soaked in water for at least an hour, then drained*
½   *cup chia seed*
1   *red bell pepper, chopped*
1   *medium carrot, chopped*
¼   *cup nutritional yeast*
     Juice of 1 lemon
     2 tablespoons miso paste
     Salt to taste
Optional: Black pepper or paprika
Optional: 1 teaspoon maple syrup for sweetness

1. Place all the ingredients into the bowl of a food processor or high-power blender (such as a Vitamix or Blendtec). Pulse until smooth and transfer to a bowl.

2. Store any uneaten portion in a tightly closed container in the refrigerator.

COCONUT PRODUCTS DEMYSTIFIED

As people become more and more savvy about the many health benefits of coconut, more and more products that feature this superfood are appearing on health food-store shelves. Here is what is currently available:

- **Coconut oil** is the nutritious oil extracted from fresh coconut meat. Rich in medium-chain fatty acids and phytonutrients, the oil's high smoke point make it fantastic for cooking. It's also great used as a flavoring and as a hair and skin moisturizer. When buying coconut oil, look for virgin coconut oil, which is obtained through cold-pressing instead of chemical extraction.

- **Coconut flour** is the finely ground, dried coconut that is left over after extracting coconut oil. Low-carbohydrate, high fiber, and gluten-free, coconut flour is a darling in the world of wheat-free baking.

- **Coconut water** is the clear liquid found inside young, green coconuts. Much touted for its amazing ability to replace electrolytes, coconut water is the natural alternative to chemical-laden sports drinks.

- **Coconut milk** is the meat of the nut blended with water to make a creamy, dairy-like liquid. Once upon a time, all coconut milk came in cans. Now, however, many brands offer cartons of coconut milk in the refrigerated dairy section of your local supermarket or health food store.

- **Dried coconut milk** is coconut milk that has been dried to a powder, much like dried milk powder. To reconstitute it, simply add milk. It's a handy, shelf-stable ingredient that can be sprinkled directly into soups and curries.

- **Coconut cream** is what many people call the thickened, creamy-looking mixture that sits at the top of a can of coconut milk.

- **Cream of coconut** goes by many names, including creamed coconut, coconut butter, coconut paste, coconut concentrate, and more. This luxurious product is literally a block or jar of thick, shortening-like coconut made from pulverized coconut flesh and oil.

- **Desiccated coconut** is a baker's favorite! Dried, unsweetened coconut is finely ground for use in cookies, cakes, breads, and other recipes. Don't confuse it with the "sweetened flaked coconut" on store shelves.

- **Coconut flakes or chips** are related to desiccated unsweetened coconut, only with bigger flakes.

- **Coconut nectar** is a low-glycemic sweetener made from the sap of coconut trees. Though it does not have a coconut-y flavor, it is rich in amino acids, minerals, and vitamins. Use it wherever you would use honey or maple syrup.
- **Coconut vinegar** is similar to apple cider vinegar, except it's made with coconut water. It is rich in electrolytes and enzymes.
- **Coconut aminos** are a blend of 17 amino acids, which are harvested from coconut trees and mixed with mineral-rich sea salt. The dark liquid is used as a replacement for soy sauce.
- **Coconut yogurt** is simply yogurt made with fermented coconut milk instead of fermented cow, sheep, or goat milk. It is a terrific choice for anyone who is allergic to dairy products.
- **Coconut keefir**, like its cousin, coconut yogurt, is nothing more than a fermented "yogurt" drink made with coconut milk instead of dairy milk.

CHIA-COCONUT SPREAD

MAKES ¾ CUPS

Rich, slightly sweet, and immensely satisfying, this nutritious spread can be slathered on bread and crackers, used as a dip, spooned onto pancakes and waffles, even thinned with oil and vinegar and revamped into a salad dressing. This is one recipe you'll come back to again and again.

½ cup creamed coconut, sometimes known as coconut cream concentrate or coconut paste, (such as Nutiva Coconut Manna, Tropicale Traditions Coconut Cream Concentrate, Let's Do Organic Creamed Coconut, or Coconut Tree's Organic Raw Coconut Crème)

3 tablespoons nut butter (cashew, almond, peanut, sunflower, etc.)

3 tablespoons chia gel (see recipe, page 77)

2 tablespoons virgin coconut oil

1 teaspoon maple syrup (or honey or agave, if desired)

1. Place the creamed coconut, nut butter, chia gel, coconut oil, and maple syrup in the bowl of a food processor or high-power blender (such as a Vitamix or Blendtec). Pulse until smooth.

2. Store any uneaten portion in a tightly closed container in the refrigerator.

CHIA QUESADILLAS

SERVES 1 OR 2

For many kids in Mexico and the western United States, quesadillas are the quintessential afterschool snack, served hot off the griddle by doting abuelas or quickly fixed by older siblings. Quesadillas are easy to make and endlessly versatile—fill them with absolutely anything you've got in your fridge!

2   8-inch corn, flour or multi-grain tortillas

⅓ cup shredded Monterey Jack or other mild cheese
1   tablespoon chia seeds
Optional: up to ⅓ cup cooked beans, fresh or frozen corn kernels, or diced, cooked vegetables
Optional: Salsa, guacamole or hot sauce for garnish

1. Place one tortilla in a large frying pan and top with the cheese, chia seeds, and filling. Place the second tortilla on top to create a sandwich.

THE SEXIEST SUPERFOOD

While the lush, rich texture of avocados makes them a darling in the culinary world, they are also prized for a staggering array of health-boosting benefits. Here are just a few of the reasons you should make avocados part of your weekly diet:

- Avocados are a powerful anti-inflammatory food, boasting a range of phytosterols, carotenoids, antioxidants, omega-3 fatty acids, and polyhydroxylated fatty acids, all of which help prevent or lessen arthritis joint afflictions, cardiovascular disease, and auto-immune disease.
- Avocados help the body absorb other nutrients. For instance, one cup of fresh avocado when eaten with a salad or other food, can increase the body's absorption of carotenoids from that food between 200 to 400 percent.
- One cup of avocado supplies 30 percent of the daily recommendation of fiber.
- Avocado has been found to help prevent the occurrence of cancers of the mouth, skin, and prostate gland, probably due to its antioxidant boosting ability and it's high content of anti-inflammatory nutrients.
- One cup of avocado has over 35 percent of one's daily allowance for vitamin K, a vitamin associated with bone formation and proper blood clotting, as well as the transport of calcium through the body.
- Individuals with latex allergies should limit their avocado consumption or avoid it completely. Unfortunately, the fruit contains high amounts of chitinase enzymes, which are associated with latex allergies. Lightly cooking the food slightly deactivates these enzymes.

2. Turn on the heat to medium-low.

3. Turn the quesadilla when the cheese begins to melt and the bottom tortilla is starting to become golden, about 3 minutes.

4. Cook on the other side for about 3 minutes.

5. Allow the quesadilla to cool slightly before cutting into wedge-shaped slices.

6. Garnish with salsa, guacamole, or hot sauce, if desired.

CHIA GUACAMOLE
MAKES ¾ CUP

Full of brain-benefiting and heart-helping monounsaturated fatty acids, guacamole is an irresistible way to get the good fats your body needs to thrive. Here, chia gel makes this wonderful food even more super. Serve it with veggie sticks, tortilla chips, quesadillas, or any other side dish that strikes your fancy.

1   avocado, preferably Hass, pitted and peeled
¼   cup chia gel (see recipe, page 77)
1   tablespoon lemon or lime juice
*   Salt, to taste*
Optional: 1 tablespoon minced red onion or
*   scallions*
Optional: A dash of hot sauce

1. In a small bowl, mash the avocado, chia gel, lemon juice, salt, and (if using) onion and hot sauce, until smooth. Serve immediately.

SOFT PRETZELS
MAKES 8 PRETZELS

Making pretzels at home is one of those "great to do with kids" activities that is easy and fun for grownups, too. This tasty recipe is so simple that you'll find yourself making it again and again.

*   Vegetable oil, for greasing pans*
1   package (or 2 ¼ teaspoons) active dry yeast
1¾ cups of barely warm water
1   tablespoon sugar or honey
4   cups whole wheat flour, plus more as needed
½   cup chia seeds
1   teaspoon salt
Optional: 1 egg, beaten, for glazing
Optional: 1 tablespoon coarse kosher salt for
*   coating*

1. Preheat oven to 425°F. Lightly oil two baking sheets.

2. In a small bowl, combine the yeast, water, and sugar. Mix thoroughly to dissolve yeast and let stand 10 minutes.

3. In a large bowl, combine the flour, chia seeds, and salt. Whisk to combine.

4. Add the yeast mixture (which should now look bubbly) to the flour mixture, stirring with a wooden spoon until stiff. When the dough is too stiff to stir, knead until it is smooth and elastic, adding small amounts of additional flour if needed to prevent stickiness.

5. Pinch off small bits of dough the size of a walnut, and roll into ropes about ¼ to ½-inch in diameter. Fashion these ropes into pretzels or other shapes, gently positioning on baking sheet. Continue until all dough has been rolled and shaped.

6. If using the glaze, brush the tops of pretzels with egg, and then sprinkle with salt.

7. Bake until the pretzels are puffy and golden, 12 to 15 minutes.

SEED COATS

Many baked goods—from artisanal breads to New York City's beloved "everything bagels"—feature a coating of mixed seeds that provide crunch, taste, and texture. If you're a baker, consider adding chia to your mixed-seed combos—it's an easy way to boost the nutrition of anything you eat.

DINNER

CHIA MEATLOAF
SERVES 6

Everyone claims to have the best meatloaf. But is it the best tasting *and* the healthiest meatloaf? This recipe can justifiably make that claim. Chia is magical in ground meat dishes. It creates a wonderful moistness and lightness, helps cut fat, increases fiber, and adds so many powerful nutrients to every bite.

½ cup beef, chicken, or vegetable broth
1 cup cooked white beans or lentils, mashed
½ cup finely chopped onion
½ cup finely chopped celery
2 cloves garlic, minced
1 teaspoon salt, or to taste
Black pepper, to taste
Vegetable oil, for greasing the pan
⅓ cup chia seeds
2 large eggs, lightly beaten
1½ pounds ground beef, or a mixture of beef and pork, turkey, or chicken

1. In a large bowl, combine the broth, mashed beans, onions, celery, garlic, salt, and pepper. Stir until well until combined.

2. Add the chia seeds and stir. Set the mixture aside for 15 minutes.

3. Preheat the oven to 350°F. Lightly oil a 5 x 9-inch loaf pan. For a free-form loaf, use a lightly oiled baking sheet.

4. Gently stir eggs into vegetable-broth-chia mixture.

5. Add the ground meat, and gently yet thoroughly combine the ingredients.

6. Pat the mixture into the loaf pan, or form into an oblong loaf shape on the prepared baking sheet. Cover the pan or baking sheet with aluminum foil.

7. Bake until golden and bubbly, about 1½ hours. (For a golden crust, remove the foil for the last 5 to 10 minutes of baking). Cool in the loaf pan for at least 15 minutes before slicing.

CHIA MEATBALLS

Love meatballs? Here's an easy, delicious, healthy way to make them: Follow the meatloaf recipe above, adding any herbs or spices you would like to the vegetable mixture. Then shape into balls (the size is up to you) and bake them on a lightly oiled baking sheet, at 350°F, until set and golden brown, about 15 minutes. Serve with marinara sauce, sweet-and-sour sauce, or your favorite gravy.

CHIA VEGETARIAN CHILI

MAKES 4 TO 6 SERVINGS

Here's yet another easy, nutritious, versatile recipe. If you don't have black beans, use white. Have leftover meat or poultry in the fridge? Chop it up and stir it in. Want to add mushrooms? Go ahead.

¼ cup olive oil
2 cups chopped onions
1⅔ cups coarsely chopped red bell peppers
    (about 2 medium)
1 cup corn kernels, fresh or frozen
6 garlic cloves, chopped
2 tablespoons chili powder
2 teaspoons dried oregano
1½ teaspoons ground cumin
½ teaspoon cayenne pepper
1 15-ounce can black beans, drained
1 15-ounce can red, pink or kidney beans,
    drained, reserving ½ cup liquid from the can

1 cup vegetable, chicken or beef broth
1 16-ounce can pureed tomatoes
½ cup chia gel (see recipe, page 77)
Optional: 1 to 2 teaspoons lime juice
Optional: 1 tablespoon cilantro, chopped
    Salt to taste

1. Heat the oil in heavy large pot over medium-high heat.
2. Add the onions, bell peppers, corn and garlic. Sauté until the onions soften, about 10 minutes.
3. Mix in the chili powder, oregano, cumin, and cayenne. Stir for 2 minutes.
4. Mix in the beans, the reserved bean liquid, broth, and the tomatoes.
5. Bring the chili to a boil, stirring occasionally.
6. Reduce the heat to medium-low and simmer until flavors blend and chili thickens, stirring occasionally, about 15 minutes.
7. Turn off heat and stir in the chia gel, lime juice, and cilantro (if using) and salt.

BENEFITS WITH BITE

Many ancient cultures used hot seasonings. In Mexico and Central America (chia's home), chili pepper was the ingredient used most often to spice up food—and, thanks to the pepper's high vitamin C, B6, and vitamin A content—it is useful in treating a variety of health conditions, including viral and bacterial infections and even cancer. The capsaicin in chilies also helps relieve muscle pain.

CHIA COTTAGE PIE

MAKES 6 SERVINGS

Back in the 1790s, recipes for cottage pies used leftover roasted meat of any kind—primarily beef—and the pie dish was lined and topped with mashed potatoes. In the 1870s, recipes for Shepherd's Pie, which featured mutton, began to appear in cookbooks, and since then it has been used synonymously with Cottage Pie.

To make Shepherd's Pie, replace all or some of the beef in this recipe with ground or minced lamb, and switch in parsnips and sweet potatoes for the Yukon Golds and lentils.

Now you have two delicious options for making, easy, savory pies.

1   *tablespoon extra-virgin olive oil*
1   *large onion, chopped*
1   *large carrot, peeled and chopped*
2   *garlic cloves, minced*
1   *pound ground beef (or substitute half or more with lamb)*
1   *cup beef or chicken broth*
1   *tablespoon tomato paste or ketchup*
1   *cup cooked lentils*
1   *teaspoon chopped fresh or dry rosemary*
1   *tablespoon chopped Italian parsley*
1   *cup frozen peas*
½   *cup chia gel (see recipe, page 77)*
2   *pounds Yukon Gold potatoes (or use regular russet potatoes) peeled and cut into chunks*
6   *tablespoons extra-virgin olive oil, virgin coconut oil or unsalted butter*
½   *cup milk (dairy, coconut, almond, rice, hemp, etc.)*
    Salt to taste

1. Preheat the oven to 375°F.

2. Heat the oil in a large sauté pan over medium-high heat, then add the onions, carrots, garlic, and meat. Cook until browned, 8 to 10 minutes.

3. Drain the excess fat from the skillet and add the broth, tomato paste, lentils, and herbs. Simmer until the juices thicken, about 10 minutes.

4. Stir in the peas and chia gel.

5. Pour the mixture into a 1½-quart baking dish; set aside

6. Meanwhile, in a saucepan, cover the potatoes with cold water and a generous pinch of salt and bring to the boil over medium-high heat. Cook until tender, about 20 minutes; drain.

7. Mash the potatoes with the oil or butter, milk, and salt.

8. Spread the potatoes over the meat mixture, then crosshatch the top with a fork.

9. Bake until golden, 30 to 35 minutes. Let stand 10 minutes before serving.

THE STORY OF PIE

"Pie...a word whose meaning has evolved in the course of many centuries and which varies to some extent according to the country or even to region. The derivation of the word may be from magpie, shortened to pie. The explanation offered in favor or this is that the magpie collects a variety of things, and that it was an essential feature of early pies that they contained a variety of ingredients. Early pies were large; but one can now apply the name to something small, as the small pork pies or mutton pies.... Early pies had pastry tops, but modern pies may have a topping of something else...or even be topless. If the basic concept of a pie is taken to mean a mixture of ingredients encased and cooked in pastry, then proto-pies were made in the classical world and pies certainly figured in early Arab cookery."

—*The Oxford Companion to Food*,
Alan Davidson (Oxford University Press, 2006)

CHIA POLENTA WITH WHITE BEANS

MAKES 4 SERVINGS

Polenta is pure comfort food. Here, it is made nutrient dense with chia and white beans. Protein, vitamins, minerals, omegas, fiber—all in one amazing-tasting dish.

2   cups stone ground cornmeal
2   cups chicken, vegetable or beef broth
1   tablespoon extra-virgin olive oil
    Salt to taste
½   cup chia gel (see recipe, page 77)
1   15-ounce can white beans
Optional garnish: Chopped tomato, minced basil, chopped scallion, marinara sauce, toasted pine nuts, chopped cooked chicken, etc.

1. In a large heavy pot over low heat, whisk together the cornmeal and broth, whisking continuously until mixture is completely lump-free.

2. Add the oil and salt, if using. Increase the heat to medium-high, stirring continuously until mixture comes to a rolling boil, about 10 minutes.

3. Lower the heat and cook, stirring continuously, for another five minutes.

4. Remove from the heat and stir in the chia gel.

5. In a small pan, warm white beans over medium-low heat.

6. To serve, spoon the polenta into shallow bowls or onto dinner plates. Top with ¼ cup of beans. Garnish as desired.

CHIA BREAKFAST POLENTA

For a warming breakfast, follow the recipe for Chia Polenta with White Beans on page 105, replacing the broth with your choice of milk (dairy, coconut, almond, rice, or hemp, etc.). Replace the olive oil with coconut oil, and omit the white beans. Garnish the cooked polenta with chopped pecans, sunflower seeds, pumpkin seeds or fruit, and a drizzle of maple syrup.

CHIA FAUX ENCHILADAS

MAKES 4 TO 6 SERVINGS

In truth, this fun recipe is more of a suggestion than a bona fide recipe. Combine the ingredients as desired—you'll get a delicious, nutritious dish each time you make these easy enchiladas. Have all ingredients at room temperature before starting.

1   *15-ounce can black or red beans*
¼   *cup chia gel (see recipe, page 77)*
1   *tablespoon extra-virgin olive oil or coconut oil*
1   *onion, sliced*
2   *red, yellow or green bell peppers, cut into narrow strips*
2   *cups protein (can be chopped meat, ground beef/pork/chicken/turkey/bison, tofu, or flaked fish)*
    Salt, to taste
1 to 2 *teaspoons lime juice*
1   *cup prepared enchilada or ranchero sauce, or salsa*
Optional: 2 tablespoons pepitas
Optional: 1 tablespoon cilantro, minced
6   *large flour, whole grain, or corn tortillas*

1. Warm the beans in a small pot over low heat. Stir in the chia gel.

2. Heat the oil in a large frying pan over medium-high heat. Add the onions and sauté for about two minutes.

3. Add the bell pepper slices to the pan. Sauté until slightly softened, about five minutes.

4. Turn off heat and add the protein, salt and lime. Stir until combined.

5. Place one tortilla on each place. Spoon one or two tablespoons of bean-chia mixture in the middle of each tortilla. Add two tablespoons of the vegetable-protein mixture.

6. Roll each tortilla, placing them seam-side down on the plate.

7. Top each faux enchilada with enchilada sauce or salsa. Garnish with pepitas and cilantro, if desired.

PEPITAS

Pepitas are green, meaty, addictive nuggets that are rich in minerals. Grown from a special variety of pumpkin that produces shell-less seeds, pepitas are high in zinc, manganese, magnesium, phosphorus, tryptophan, and iron. They also contain high doses of protein, vitamin K, and fiber. For a fun snack, dry toast pepitas in a clean pan until they pop, then dress them with salt and a dusting of chili powder or a splash of soy sauce.

CHIA CHIPOTLE BEAN BURGER

MAKES 4 TO 6 SERVINGS

Bean burgers make a fast, casual, and tasty meal that is high in protein and fiber, and low in fat. Go ahead and make this recipe your own: Play around with the veggies and seasonings and experiment with other types of beans—you can use kidney and cannellini beans, chickpeas, or even lentils.

1   *15-ounce can black beans*
¼   *cup chia gel (see recipe, page 77)*
2   *cloves garlic, minced*
¼   *cup corn kernels or sautéed or cooked*
    vegetables (alternatively, use frozen corn
    kernels, defrosted, or vegetables leftover
    from another meal)
1   *teaspoon canned chipotle in adobo, minced,*
    or 1 teaspoon dried chipotle powder

½   *teaspoon salt*
Optional: 1 tablespoon minced cilantro or
    parsley
1   *tablespoon virgin coconut oil*

1. In the bowl of a food processor or high-speed blender (such as a Vitamix or Blendtec), pulse the ingredients until blended. Do not over-process; you do not want to liquefy!
2. Form the mixture into patties.
3. Heat the coconut oil in a frying pan over medium heat.
4. Cook the patties until golden, about five minutes. Flip and repeat.
5. Alternate cooking method: Preheat oven to 325°F. Place the patties on a lightly oiled baking sheet and cook until golden, 12 to 15 minutes, turning halfway through cooking.
6. Serve on hamburger rolls with the condiments of your choice.

BLACK BEAUTIES

Black beans are well known in nutrition circles for their high fiber content. In fact, black beans have more fiber than the other legume powerhouses—lentils and chickpeas. The fiber in these treasures has been shown to be perfect for helping the lower digestive tract stay healthy, lowering the risk of colon cancer and helping to create efficient digestion.

CHIA CHICKEN BURGERS
MAKES 6 TO 8 SERVINGS

Ground chicken is a terrific option for anyone who is trying to lower their red meat consumption. It's also fantastic for dieters, containing approximately 50 percent less calories than ground pork or beef. In this recipe, ground chicken and chia team up to make the most tender, moist burgers you're ever likely to eat.

2   pounds ground white meat chicken
    (or dark meat, although it contains more
    calories and fat than white chicken meat)
2   tablespoons chia gel (see recipe, page 77)
1 or 2 garlic cloves, minced
    Salt and black pepper, to taste
Optional: 1 to 2 tablespoons minced fresh
    parsley, chives, or a mix of these, and any
    other fresh herb of your choice
1   tablespoon extra-virgin olive oil or virgin
    coconut oil

1. In large bowl, mix together the ground chicken, chia gel, garlic, salt, black pepper, and fresh herbs, if using, combining gently yet thoroughly.
2. Form the meat mixture into 6 to 8 patties, about ¾-inch thick.
3. Add the oil to a large frying pan over medium heat. Cook the patties on one side, until browned, 7 to 8 minutes. Turn, and continue cooking until cooked through completely, about 6 minutes more. Serve on hamburger rolls with the condiments of your choice.

GROUND CHICKEN VS. GROUND BEEF

Anyone who is watching their calories knows that ground beef is rich in calories. A 4-ounce serving of ground beef has roughly 250 calories. You can lighten your favorite recipes by swapping in ground chicken. It contains only 130 calories per 4-ounce serving.

CHIA CAESAR SALAD
MAKES 2 SERVINGS

Caesar salad is the quintessential restaurant salad, the go-to item when you want something light (yet filling), healthy, and delicious. This quick, at-home version tastes just like what you'd get at your favorite restaurant, except it doesn't contain eggs or anchovies, and we've left off the croutons to create a lower-calorie dish. Also, there's plenty of chia in this Caesar salad to raise its fiber and nutrient profile.

2 or 3 Romaine hearts, leaves washed, dried
    and chopped, or torn into bite-sized pieces
⅓ cup extra-virgin olive oil
2   tablespoons chia gel (see recipe, page 77)
    Juice of 1 lemon
1   teaspoon Tabasco sauce
1   teaspoon Worcestershire sauce
1   teaspoon Dijon mustard
1 or 2 garlic cloves, minced
¼ cup Parmesan cheese, grated
    Salt and freshly ground black pepper, to taste

1. Place the chopped romaine in a salad bowl.

2. In a blender, pulse the remaining ingredients until liquefied.

3. Toss the salad with dressing, using only enough to coat lettuce. Store the remaining dressing in a tightly closed container in the refrigerator and use within a week.

SUPER CAESER

If the stories are true, Caesar salad is the creation of Caesar Cardini, who owned restaurants in the United States and Mexico. According to his daughter Rosa, Cardini invented the famous salad in the kitchen of his San Diego restaurant on the Fourth of July, 1924, when a rush on the kitchen depleted supplies. While the original version featured plenty of croutons, it did not use anchovies. If you'd like, add white meat chicken or turkey to your salad for a well-rounded meal.

CHIA GAZPACHO
MAKES 8 SERVINGS

Homemade gazpacho is one of life's great pleasures. Many of us can't imagine summer without it. This savory recipe uses white chia seed, for thickening, instead of the more traditional bread crumbs.

1   46-ounce can or jar of tomato juice
2   cups vegetable or chicken broth
2   cups finely chopped fresh plum tomatoes
½   cup finely chopped yellow or red bell pepper
½   cup peeled, seeded finely chopped cucumber
½   cup finely chopped red or sweet onion (such as Maui, Walla Walla, or Vidalia)
¼   cup red wine vinegar
¼   cup white chia seeds
⅓   cup extra-virgin olive oil
    Juice of ½ lemon
¼   cup minced parsley, or a combination of parsley and chives
1   teaspoon fresh oregano, minced
2   cloves garlic, minced
    Salt, to taste
    Black pepper, to taste
    Hot sauce, to taste
Optional garnish: chopped parsley or chives, minced red or sweet onion, chopped olives, pepitas, or anything else that sounds delicious

1. In a large bowl, combine all the ingredients, except salt, pepper, hot sauce, and garnish. Mix thoroughly.

2. Taste and season with salt, pepper, and hot sauce.

3. Refrigerate at least 2 hours before serving. The soup will thicken as the chia seed swells.

4. Serve with optional garnish.

DESSERTS

BASIC CHIA PUDDING

MAKES 3 TO 4 SERVINGS

This is dessert at its easiest—just mix chia seeds with your a favorite liquid, sweeten it, allow it to stand and thicken, then serve it as-is—or with nuts, sugar, fruit, shaved chocolate, or anything else that strikes your fancy.

2   *cups almond milk (can also use coconut, rice, hemp, or dairy milk)*
¾   *cup chia seeds*
2   *tablespoons honey or maple syrup*
     Dash salt
Optional: vanilla or almond extract, to taste

1. In a large bowl, mix all the ingredients together, stirring well to combine. Allow pudding to sit for five minutes, and then stir again.

2. Give the pudding a stir every five minutes over a 30-minute period, until the pudding is thickened.

3. Pudding will be ready when the chia seeds have plumped up.

4. Refrigerator until ready to serve.

CACAO VS. COCOA

Cacao is made of the solids left behind after the liqueur and butter have been removed from the cacao beans. There is loud, frequent debate among foodies about the difference between cacao and cocoa powders. In truth, there is no difference, other than the spelling. If you come across the word "raw" tacked onto cacao powder, it simply means that the product has not been heated above 110°F.

CACAO-CHIA PUDDING

MAKES 2 SERVINGS

Deep and intense, this chocolaty dessert is rich in magnesium, iron, zinc, and many other powerful nutrients.

2½ cups water
1 cup raw cashews
5 chopped soft, pitted dates (soak in hot water for an hour if dates are hard)
2 tablespoons vanilla extract
  Dash salt
½ cup raw cacao powder (or cacao nibs or regular unsweetened natural cocoa powder)
⅓ cup chia seed

1. In a food processor or high-power blender (such as a Vitamix or Blendtec), process the water, cashews, dates, vanilla extract, and salt. Pulse until absolutely smooth.
2. Add the cacao powder and chia, and blend just until smooth.
3. Pour into dessert cups and refrigerate overnight until firm.

BERRY CLOUD PUDDING

MAKES 2 TO 4 SERVINGS

This brilliant pink dessert tastes like summer. It's a light, refreshing way to end a meal—but it also makes a special snack or a dressy brunch option. Go ahead and experiment with different fruit and flavorings.

2 cups frozen or fresh strawberries or raspberries (or a combination)
⅔ cup canned coconut milk, shaken before measuring (do not use "lite" coconut milk)
2 tablespoons milled chia seed (see recipe, page 71)
1 to 2 tablespoons honey, to taste
1 tablespoon lemon or lime juice
  Splash vanilla, almond, or lemon extract

1. Place all the ingredients in a high-power blender, such as a Vitamix or Blendtec and blend until combined and berry seeds have been pulverized.
2. Pour the pudding into 2 to 4 dessert cups and refrigerate about 2 hours, or until cold and set.

CHIA ICE POPS

MAKES 4 TO 6 SERVINGS

Popsicles are a great place to experiment with chia, milled chia, and chia gel. This fruity, refreshing recipe uses whole strawberries, mango chunks, and orange juice, but feel free to experiment. The combinations are—quite literally—endless.

1 cup frozen strawberries
1 cup frozen mango chunks
½ cup orange juice
⅓ cup chia seeds
¼ cup water

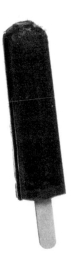

1. In a food processor or high-power blender (such as Vitamix or Blendtec), blend all the ingredients until liquefied.
2. Pour into ice pop molds or ice cube molds.
3. Freeze until solid.

INVENTING THE POPSICLE

- The first popsicle was created in 1905 by an 11-year-old boy named Frank Epperson, who called his invention the Epsicle Ice Pop.
- Epperson invented the treat after leaving a cup of soda with a straw outdoors during the winter. It froze—and Epperson had himself a frozen treat.
- It took Epperson more than 18 years to finally patent his invention. By that time, his own children had taken to calling the treats "popsicles." The new name stuck.
- In 1925, Epperson sold the rights to his popsicle to the John Lowe food company of New York.
- The first commercial popsicles had birch sticks. Today, most popsicle sticks are still made of birch.

CHIA GELATIN

MAKES ABOUT 4 SERVINGS

This textured dessert does not resemble the smooth, neon-colored, rubbery dessert you may remember from childhood. Chia gelatin is full of bumpy, nutty chia seeds, and is a deeply nourishing comfort food. For a creamier dessert, use coconut milk instead of fruit juice (or combine them).

3¾ cup fruit juice of your choice
¼ cup chia seeds
1 15-ounce container coconut milk (this needs to be cold) or additional fruit juice
4 envelopes powdered gelatin (Knox brand)

1. Mix ¾ cup of the fruit juice and the chia seeds in a small bowl. Let sit for 3 minutes and stir again. Place the bowl in the fridge for 1 to 2 hours until the mixture becomes firm.
2. In a medium saucepan or pot, heat the remaining 3 cups of fruit juice.
3. While the juice is heating, sprinkle the gelatin over the cold coconut milk in a small bowl and let it stand while the juice on the stove heats to a boil.
4. In an 8-inch x 11-inch glass baking-dish, mix the boiling juice and the coconut milk-gelatin mixture, whisking for about five minutes until there are no lumps and everything is dissolved.
5. Take the chia-juice mixture out of the fridge.
6. When the gelatin mixture has cooled down, for 10 or 15 minutes, add a tablespoon of the chia mixture to the gelatin mixture, whisking until combined. Continue adding small amounts of chia mixture to gelatin mixture, stirring after each addition, until finished.
7. Place in the refrigerator until set.

THE FACTS ABOUT GELATIN

Unflavored gelatin (a key ingredient in JELL-O®) is in fact an animal product that confers a number of excellent health benefits. In the autism community, for example, it is a popular remedy to help heal leaky gut syndrome (where the walls of the large intestine are porous), and studies have also found gelatin to be helpful in treating joint and tendon conditions.

RAW CHIA-CACAO COOKIES

MAKES ABOUT 12 SMALL COOKIES

For many of us, these cookies are the ultimate, high protein, high nutrient, completely raw cookie—nothing like the Toll House sweets of our youth. You'll love the energy you get from these yummy treats.

1   *cup pitted dates*
½   *cup raw slivered almonds*
2   *tablespoons raw cacao powder (or cacao nibs or regular unsweetened natural cocoa powder)*
⅛   *cup chia seeds*
1   *teaspoon vanilla*
¼   *cup whole raw cashews, hazelnuts, pistachios, or almonds*

1. Using a food processor or a high-power blender (such as a Vitamix or Blendtec), process the dates until a smooth paste forms.
2. Add the almonds, cacao powder, chia seeds, and vanilla. Pulse until everything is combined, but not liquefied.
3. Add the raw cashews and pulse only until the nuts are incorporated into the mix—you want chunky pieces of nut distributed throughout the cookies.
4. Roll tablespoon-sized balls of dough between your hands to make a perfectly round, smoothly-finished cookie.
5. Place the cookies on a piece of waxed paper to firm up for at least 2 hours. Store in the refrigerator or freezer.

RAW CACAO NIBS

If you're a hardcore raw food enthusiast, the thought of using anything but raw cacao may pain you. If you can't find raw cacao powder, simply use an equal amount of raw cacao nibs, and pulverize them into a soft powder.

NUT BUTTER CHIA COOKIES

MAKES 20 TO 24 COOKIES

These pretty little cakes are akin to the peanut butter cookies you grew up on—but they're loaded with protein and fiber. To make the cookies gluten free, try using gluten-free oat flour. The cookies will be a touch softer and more fragile than traditional peanut butter cookies, but they're every bit as delicious.

½   *cup virgin coconut oil*
½   *cup natural cane sugar (e.g., Sucanat) or regular granulated sugar*
½   *cup brown sugar*
½   *cup unsalted cashew butter (can also use almond butter)*
1   *large egg*
1   *teaspoon vanilla extract*
1¼ *cups oat flour or whole-wheat pastry flour*
¼   *cup ground almond meal*
3   *tablespoons chia seeds*
¾   *teaspoon baking soda*
½   *teaspoon fine grain sea salt*

1. Preheat the oven to 350°F. Prepare two baking sheets by lining with parchment paper.

2. Using a stand mixer, beat together the coconut oil, sugars, and cashew butter for about 4 or 5 minutes, or until light in color.

3. Add the egg and vanilla, beating just until completely blended.

4. In a medium bowl, whisk together the flour, almond meal, chia seeds, baking soda, and salt. Add the flour mixture to the wet ingredients, mixing just until blended.

5. Using a tablespoon or a medium-size cookie scoop, drop batter onto lined baking sheets. Press down gently on the cookies with the tines of a fork or use a glass tumbler to flatten them slightly.

6. Bake until golden brown, 12 to 15 minutes.

7. Cool for 1 to 2 minutes before removing the cookies from the pans.

MAKING YOUR OWN OAT AND ALMOND FLOUR

Although you can easily buy oat or almond flour at a specialty or health food store—they can be made just as easily at home. To make oat flour, simply whir the oats in a coffee grinder or food processor. To make almond flour, you can use raw or toasted almonds, just be sure to pulse the nuts carefully so that you don't over-process them. The texture of the flour should be sand-like.

WALNUT SPONGE CAKE
MAKES 12 SERVINGS

This elegant cake is based on a recipe by Vilma Lo Presti, which you can find in her magnificent chia cookbook, *Pastrymaking and Baking with Chia* (De Los Cuatrovientos, 2009). The directions are a bit involved, but when you really want to impress, you'll be happy you took the time to make this amazing cake!

6   *large egg whites, divided*
1   *large egg*
⅔   *cup granulated sugar, divided*
2½ *tablespoons honey*
3½ *tablespoons virgin coconut oil, plus more*
    for greasing pan
½   *teaspoon cream of tartar*
1   *cup cake flour*
⅔   *cup whole wheat pastry flour, plus more*
    for dusting pan
2   *teaspoons baking powder*
⅓   *cup walnuts, finely chopped*
5   *tablespoon milled chia (see recipe, page 71)*
Optional topping: Confectioner's sugar

1. Preheat oven to 325°F. Prepare an 8-inch cake pan by lightly oiling and dusting with flour. Set aside.

2. In the bowl of a standing mixer, using the whisk attachment, beat two of the egg whites and the whole egg with half the sugar and the honey until creamy.

3. With the motor on low, slowly drizzle the oil into the egg mixture. Remove the bowl and set aside.

4. Attach a fresh bowl to the mixer and beat the remaining four egg whites with the remaining sugar and the cream of tartar. Beat until the mixture forms soft, flexible peaks.

5. In a separate large bowl, sift together both flours and the baking powder.

6. With the mixer on low—or using a large spatula and working by hand, alternately fold the egg-sugar mixture and flour mixture into the whipped egg whites.

7. Gently fold in the walnuts and milled chia.

THE HEALTH BENEFITS OF WALNUTS

Walnuts are filled with good things—protein, omega-3 fatty acids, vitamin E, and manganese. Walnuts benefit the cardiovascular and immune systems, the skin, and the nervous system. Surprisingly, only 5.5 percent of American adults eat walnuts at any point during the year! Here are some more interesting facts about walnuts:

- Due to their high polyunsaturated fat content, walnuts are extremely perishable and should be stored in the refrigerator or freezer.
- In the 4th century A.D., the Romans introduced walnuts to many European countries, where they have been grown ever since.
- Walnut oil was once used as lamp oil.
- A 1-ounce serving of walnuts amounts to about 7 shelled walnuts, or 14 walnut halves.
- Walnuts are part of the tree nut family, which includes Brazil nuts, cashews, hazelnuts, macadamia nuts, pecans, pine nuts, and pistachios.
- China is the largest commercial producer of walnuts in the world, with about 360,000 metric tons produced per year.
- The United States is the second largest commercial producer of walnuts, with about 294,000 metric tons of production.
- In the United States, 90 percent of all walnuts are grown in Northern California, most notably, the Sacramento and San Joaquin valleys.
- Turkey, Iran, Ukraine, and Romania are the next highest walnut producers in the world, after California.
- The walnuts grown commercially in the U.S. are known as "English walnuts" because they were first brought to our shores on British mercantile ships.
- Black walnuts are native to the United States.

8. Pour batter into the prepared pan and place it in the oven. Bake until a toothpick inserted in the middle comes out clean, about 40 minutes.

9. Allow the cake to cool 10 minutes in the pan before inverting and cooling completely on a rack.

10. Dust with confectioner's sugar, if desired.

MOIST CARROT CAKE
MAKES 12 TO 16 SERVINGS

Carrot cakes, though popular in the United States since the 1960s, can be traced back to the carrot puddings of medieval Europe. This moist dessert is based upon a recipe created by Vilma Lo Presti. (You can find it in her magnificent chia cookbook, *Pastrymaking and Baking with Chia.*) It takes some care to prepare this delicious, moist cake, but it is so worth the effort! Omit the optional glaze and save yourself 180 calories per serving.

7   tablespoons virgin coconut oil, plus more
      for greasing pan
6   tablespoons granulated sugar
6   tablespoons packed brown sugar
1   large egg
3   large egg whites
1½ cups carrot puree, made by cooking carrots
      and mashing them or pureeing them in
      a food processor
7   tablespoons part skim ricotta cheese
1   tablespoon grated orange rind
1   cup all-purpose flour, plus more for
      dusting pan
½   cup whole wheat pastry flour
3   teaspoon baking powder
½   teaspoon cinnamon
      Dash salt
½   cup walnuts or pecans, finely chopped
⅓   cup dark seedless raisins, packed
¼   cup chia seeds

For the Glaze
1½ cups powdered sugar
6   tablespoons unsweetened cocoa powder
¼   cup dark rum

1. Preheat oven to 350°F. Lightly oil and flour a bundt pan.

2. In the bowl of a stand mixer fitted with the paddle attachment, beat the coconut oil, both sugars, and the whole egg together until creamy.

3. Add the egg whites, one by one, blending well after each addition.

4. Add carrot puree, blending thoroughly.

5. Mix in ricotta and orange rind, blending thoroughly.

6. In a separate bowl, whisk together the flours, baking powder, cinnamon, and salt.

7. Add the flour mixture to the egg-carrot mixture, mixing only until blended.

8. Gently mix in nuts, raisins, and chia, and pour the batter into the prepared pan.

CARROT TRIVIA

Who doesn't love a bit of trivia, especially when it is about food?

- The longest carrot, recorded in 1996, was 5.14 meters (16 feet 10½ inches).
- Carrots have the highest content of beta-carotene (vitamin A) of all vegetables.
- Carrots were first grown as a medicine, not a food.
- Anglo-Saxons included carrots as an ingredient in a medicinal drink to ward off the devil and insanity.
- The heaviest carrot on record, so far, weighed 18.985 pounds, and was harvested in 1998 by John V. R. Evans, an American farmer.
- Many people trace the modern carrot cake to Viola Schlicting, from Texas, who created the first carrot cake in the 1960s from her German carrot-nut bread recipe.
- Carrots were the first vegetable to be canned commercially.
- Holtville, California is known as "The Carrot Capital of the World."
- Researchers at the USDA found that study participants who consumed two carrots a day were able to lower their cholesterol levels by about 20 percent, due to the vegetable's soluble fiber.
- When juiced, one pound of carrots will make approximately 6 to 8 ounces of carrot juice.
- A teaspoon holds almost 2,000 carrot seeds.
- The last meal on the *Titanic* included creamed carrots in the fifth course.

9. Bake until golden and a toothpick inserted in the center of the cake comes out clean, 35 to 40 minutes.

10. Cool the cake in the pan for 10 to 15 minutes before inverting onto a wire rack to cool completely.

11. If using the glaze, whisk the ingredients together in a small bowl. Drizzle over the cake while it is still warm.

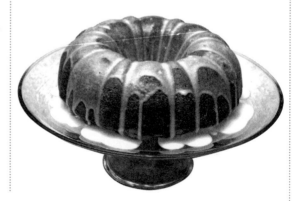

BEAUTY RECIPES

Omega-3 fatty acid is fantastic for skin, hair, and nails, making chia the ultimate beauty food. Eating chia regularly ensures you look your best, but you can also mix chia into your favorite lotions, cleansers, shampoos and conditioners to look even better. Or, be adventurous and use one of our recipes.

MOISTURIZING CHIA-AVOCADO MASK

MAKES ENOUGH FOR 1 APPLICATION

This rich mask is made for drier skin. It's ultra-moisturizing, nourishing, and firming. Use it weekly, if you'd like, and see the difference in your skin.

½ *avocado, pit removed*
1 *tablespoon milled chia seeds (see recipe, page 71)*
Optional: 1 drop of lavender essential oil

1. Scoop avocado flesh from the peel into a medium bowl.
2. Add chia seed and essential oil, if using. Mash mixture into a smooth paste.
3. Place on clean facial skin and allow to sit for 15 to 30 minutes.
4. Remove with a washcloth that has been moistened in warm water.

THE BEAUTY BOOSTER

If you're looking for a fast way to add chia seeds to your beauty routine, stir a tablespoon of milled chia or chia gel into your favorite packaged facial masque, body scrub, or hair conditioner. Allow the mixture to sit for as long as you'd like, then rinse it off. Voila!: softer skin and hair.

SQUEEZE YOUR OWN ALOE

Depending upon where you live, you may find large, single aloe leaves in the produce department of your local supermarket, health food store, or a market such as Whole Foods. If you've been relying on bottles of shelf-stable aloe vera gel from the drug store, give fresh aloe a try. Cooling, refreshing, tightening, brightening, ultra-healing, and super-nourishing, the aloe's light gel is heavenly on skin and great on hair as a light styling gel. To harvest your own, go ahead and purchase one of those leaves, looking for one that is firm and even in color. Once you bring it home, slit the leaf lengthwise and use a spoon to scoop out the clear gel.

SKIN FRESHENING MASK
MAKES ENOUGH FOR 1 APPLICATION

This light, refreshing mask is ideal for normal to oilier skin. It leaves your skin soft and glowing.

4 tablespoons raw aloe gel (from the health
    food store or squeezed from an aloe leaf)
1 tablespoon milled chia seeds (see recipe, page 71)
Optional: 1 drop of tea tree essential oil

1. Stir the ingredients together in a medium bowl.
2. Apply to clean facial skin, allowing the mixture to sit for 15 to 30 minutes.
3. Remove with a washcloth that has been moistened in warm water.

KELP FACE PACK
MAKES ENOUGH FOR 1 APPLICATION

Seaweed is a wonder for firming the skin and creating a glowing finish.

1 tablespoon powdered kelp (buy kelp at
    the health food store and whir in a coffee
    grinder)
1 tablespoon plain yogurt
1 tablespoon chia gel (see recipe, page 77)

1. Mix the ingredients in a medium bowl, stirring until combined.
2. Apply to clean facial skin, allowing the mixture to sit for 15 to 30 minutes.
3. Remove with a washcloth that has been moistened in warm water.

SEAWEED TO THE RESCUE

Seaweed is a common ingredient in high-end and health-food store skin preparations. Kelp, dulse, and wakame have similar properties to human plasma, and are also concentrated sources of many minerals (including iodine) and vitamins that leave skin nourished, soft, smooth, and radiant.

SUPER FAST FACE PACK I
MAKES ENOUGH FOR 1 APPLICATION

Speedy and nourishing, this quick recipe revives skin, giving it a vibrant look.

2 to 3 tablespoons chia gel (see recipe, page 77)

1. Apply to clean facial skin, allowing the mixture to sit for 15 to 30 minutes.
2. Remove with a washcloth that has been moistened in warm water.

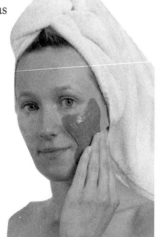

SUPER FAST FACE PACK II

MAKES ENOUGH FOR 1 APPLICATION

Here's another quick and easy way to give your skin a glow.

2   *tablespoons milled chia*
2   *tablespoons aloe gel, plain yogurt, rose water, or your favorite facial toner or facial moisturizer*

1. Mix the ingredients in a medium bowl, stirring until combined.
2. Apply to clean facial skin, allowing the mixture to sit for 15 to 30 minutes.
3. Remove with a washcloth that has been moistened in warm water.

ROSE WATER

Rose water is the by-product of the rose oil used in perfume. Rose water is used as a flavoring agent in the Middle East and Southern Europe, and it is a popular skincare ingredient in America, where it is often found in astringents and toners. These products are designed to remove traces of makeup and impurities, and leave the skin looking even-pored, firm, and fresh.

ALMOND FACE SCRUB

MAKES ENOUGH FOR 1 APPLICATION

Almond scrubs are traditional treatments

JOJOBA OIL

Jojoba oil was the skincare darling of the 1970s, showing up in massage oil, facial creams, shaving preparations, nail strengtheners, and all kinds of mainstream hair products. We still love the all-day moisture just a few small drops provide … although we must share just one interesting bit of jojoba trivia: Jojoba oil isn't really an oil at all, but the wax ester (liquid wax) of the jojoba bean.

for sloughing off dead skin and impurities to create fresh, soft skin. Try this homemade version. You'll be happily surprised at how gorgeous your skin can look.

2   *tablespoons coarse almond meal*
1   *tablespoon milled chia seeds*
1   *tablespoon jojoba oil (for drier skin) or aloe vera gel (for oilier skin)*

1. Whisk the ingredients together in a medium bowl.
2. Apply to clean facial skin, scrubbing the mixture into the skin in small circles. Pay extra attention to rough areas or areas that contain congested pores.
3. Rise immediately with warm water, or allow the mixture to sit for 10 to 30 minutes before rinsing.

HIGH GLOW SCRUB

MAKES ENOUGH TO USE ON THE BODY AND FACE

This easy recipe creates a scrub that is both nourishing and invigorating.

½ cup chia gel (see recipe, page 77)
2 to 4 tablespoons kosher or Epsom salt,
   or raw sugar crystals (such as Sucanat)
Optional: 1 drop lavender essential oil

1. Whisk the ingredients to gether in a large bowl, using a larger amount of salt or sugar for a rougher-grained scrub.
2. In the shower, rub onto dry skin, working in small circles on the body and face.
3. Allow the mixture to sit for a few minutes if desired, or rinse immediately.

CHIA NAIL TREATMENT
MAKES ENOUGH FOR 1 APPLICATION

In this recipe, chia helps freshen, strengthen, and moisturize nails.

1   teaspoon lemon juice
1   teaspoon honey
1   tablespoon milled chia (see recipe, page 71)

1. Mix the ingredients in a medium bowl, stirring until combined.
2. Apply to fingernails, rubbing into the nails, cuticles, and surrounding skin. (May also be applied to toenails in the same way.)
3. Rinse immediately, or allow the mixture to sit for 10 minutes before removing.

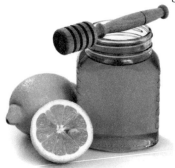

PET FOODS

Animals thrive when given a nutrient-dense diet. Upgrading your pet's health is simple with chia. Just stir into food (or sprinkle onto it) and serve. More ideas below.

CANARY CRUNCH
MAKES 2½ CUPS

This fast, easy food creates energy and a bright coat of feathers. It's perfect as a main food or snack for canaries, parakeets, parrots, love birds, cockatiels, cockatoos, doves and other exotic pet birds.

2 *cups commercial bird seed*
½ *cup chia seeds*

1. Mix together the bird seed and chia, and store in a tightly covered container in a cool spot.

SHARING THE WEALTH

Canary Crunch can also be used in bird-feeders for small birds or scattered on the ground for peacocks, swans, and other water birds. Why should domesticated birds have all the nutrients?

EGGCELLENT!

You've probably seen "omega-enriched" eggs at the supermarket. Have you ever wonder how they got to be so high in these essential fatty acids? It all starts with chicken feed. In other words, whatever hens eat a lot of, ends up in their eggs. Thus, many farmers are feeding their chickens flax or chia to increase the amount of omega-3 fatty acid in eggs. If too much flax is fed the eggs will have a fishy flavor, this is not the case with chia, however.

CHICKEN FEED
MAKES ABOUT 12 CUPS

Chia is gaining attention not only for what it can do for the chicken you eat, but for the eggs that chickens lay: Feeding birds chia seed is a fast, easy, safe way to increase the omega fatty acid content of the meat and eggs.

5 *pound bag of commercial chicken feed*
1 *pound bag of chia seeds*

1. In a large container or bucket with a lid, combine the chicken feed and chia seeds.
2. Store, covered, in a cool, dry place.

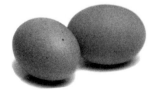

RABBIT STUDIES

In 2010, the University of Turin conducted research to determine the difference between rabbits that consumed chia and those that had not. After replacing up to 15 percent of the bunnies' regular diets with chia, researchers found no change in meat texture or taste between the two groups. However, the chia-fed rabbits had meat with higher antioxidant levels, higher omega-3 and -6 fatty acids, less saturated fat, and more unsaturated lipids (a good thing; these contribute to cardiovascular health).

BUNNY CHIA DRINK

MAKES ENOUGH FOR 1 DAY'S WATER SUPPLY

It's hard to get pet rabbits to eat chia—they aren't seed eaters, and chia doesn't stick well to the grasses, vegetables, and commercial food pellets that most domestic rabbits consume. This bunny drink is one way to get chia into your beloved pet.

1   *cup fresh water*
½   *teaspoon chia gel (see recipe, page 77)*

1. Add chia gel to water. Mix thoroughly to blend.
2. Place in a water bowl chia gel may clog a water sipper.

CHIA CAT FOOD
MAKES 1 SERVING

Chia helps cats' coats grow glossy and thick, brightens their eyes, and help sustain their energy levels.

1   *serving of canned food (depending on your cat, this is 1 ounce, 3 ounce, or 5 ounce)*
1   *teaspoon chia gel (see recipe, page 77)*

1. Mix chia gel with canned food until it's thoroughly mixed.
2. Serve immediately.

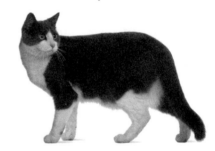

CHIA GRASS

If you're a cat owner, you've probably seen your cat chew on houseplants or grass. You may have even treated your pet with her very own pot of wheatgrass. Next time try chia grass. Chia Grass Cat Planters allow you to grow your own chia grass at home. Cats love nibbling on it—as do dogs, rabbits, guinea pigs, birds, horses, cows, sheep, and goats. You might want to get two!

CHIA DOG FOOD

MAKES ENOUGH FOR 1 SERVING

As dogs get older, their coats get dull. Some animals become prone to skin conditions, and frankly, they begin to smell on the strong side. A daily dosage of chia can help keep fur gleaming, skin supple, and odors to a minimum.

*1 serving of canned food (half or more of a
12-ounce can)*
1 tablespoon chia gel (see recipe, page 77)

1. Mix chia gel into the canned food until thoroughly mixed.
2. Serve immediately.

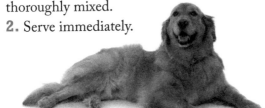

HORSE CHOW

MAKES ENOUGH FOR 1 SERVING

Omega fatty acids do wonderful thing to hair, skin, and nails—or hooves, in the case of horses. They also improve joint health, helping older animals and workhorses feel more comfortable.

⅔ cup alfalfa or grass pellets
⅓ cup chia seed

1. Place the pellets in a trough, on the ground, or in a feeder.
2. Pour chia seed on top.

LIVESTOCK FEED

MAKES 1 SERVING

This nourishing recipe is great for cows, goats, and sheep—all ruminants, a word that comes from the Latin ruminare, which means "to chew over again."

¼ cup chia seeds per each goat or sheep; 1 cup chia seeds per cow
Regular serving of hay or grain or food pellets

1. Sprinkle or pour dry chia seeds directly over the food that your animals regularly eat.

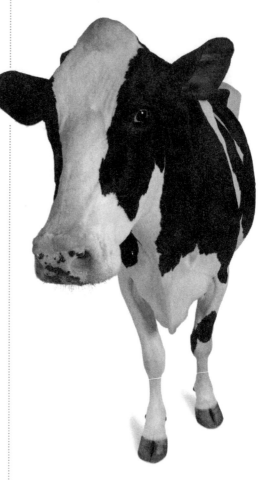

SUPER MILK

Giving chia to cows, goats, and sheep chia is an easy way to enhance the milk they produce with omega fatty acids and other nutrients found in chia seeds. Whether it is consumed as milk or made into yogurt, sour cream, cheeses, or other dairy products, this enhanced milk is becoming a popular way for the food industry to meet consumer demands for enhanced dairy products.

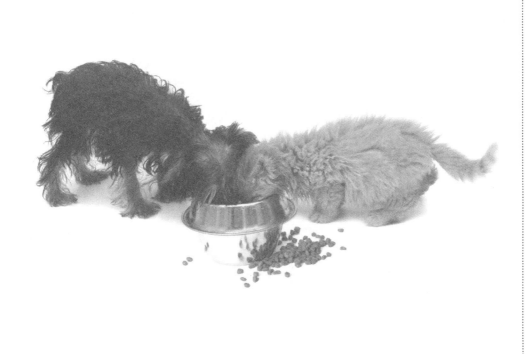

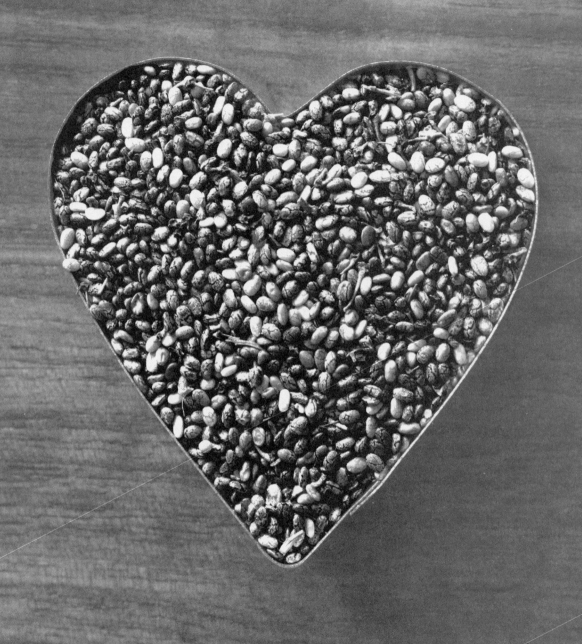

CHAPTER 6

STAYING HEALTHY WITH CHIA

One of the reasons chia is such a wonder food is that it truly does offer something to just about everyone, whether you're young, old, or middle-aged, male or female, a couch potato or an elite athlete. Chia can help you overcome illnesses and help prevent them. It can even make your hair grow better!

In other words, chia is about much more than weight loss. This chapter lets you in on all the conditions that can be helped and even prevented with a daily dose of chia.

CANCER

Regardless of the type of cancer, the condition starts when the DNA within a single cell mutates, then replicates, creating more mutated cells. Soon these fast-moving, mutating cells begin invading healthy tissue—this is how cancer spreads. This mutation can be caused by a genetic mistake or by exposure to radiation or a carcinogen. Some cancers are slow-moving, easily caught, and easily treated. Others are stealthy and fast—by the time a person knows he or she has cancer, it is almost too late.

One or two tablespoons of chia a day can help both prevent cell mutations, as well as slow already-mutating cells, making conventional cancer therapies more successful. How? It all has to do with chia's high levels of antioxidants. These phytonutrients help supercharge and protect cells from DNA damage. They also help damaged cells repair themselves. Among the cancer-fighting antioxidants in chia are: Vitamins A, C, and E, chlorogenic and caffeic acids, myricetin, quercetin, and kaempferol flavonol, chlorogenic acid, and flavonol glycosides.

Omega-3 fatty acid also helps fight and prevent cancer. In 2007, researchers at the Universidad Nacional de Córdoba, in Córdoba, Argentina, studied the effect of this fatty acid on breast cancer tumors. The findings, which were published in the July 2007 issue of *Journal of Prostaglandins, Leukotrienes and Essential Fatty Acids*, showed that the omega-3 fatty acid in chia helped shrink existing tumors and prevent metastasizing.

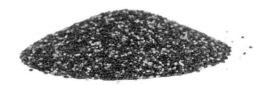

CANCER FACTS

- Lung cancer is one of the most preventable types of cancer.
- There are over 100 kinds of cancer.
- Any body part can be affected by cancer.
- A third of cancers can be cured if detected early and treated adequately.
- Tobacco use is the single largest preventable cause of cancer in the world.
- More than 70 percent of the world's cancer deaths occur in middle- and low-income countries.
- 8.4 million Americans alive today either have cancer or have had it in their past.
- Once a person quits smoking, it will take him or her 10 years to replace all the precancerous cells in his or her body.
- Worldwide, the five most common types of cancer that kill women are (in the order of frequency): breast, lung, stomach, colorectal, and cervical.
- Remission is a sign that cancer cells may have already been eliminated.
- Not all cancers develop into tumors.
- When cancer cells spread to other parts of the body, it is called metastasis.
- Symptoms of cancer are: weight loss, tiredness, or exhaustion, fever, and swollen glands.
- Worldwide, the five most common cancers among men are (in order of frequency): lung, stomach, liver, colorectal, and esophagus.
- One-fifth of all cancers worldwide are caused by a chronic infection. For example, the human papillomavirus (HPV) causes cervical cancer and the hepatitis B virus (HBV) causes liver cancer.
- The most common cancers diagnosed in the Unites States are: bladder cancer, breast cancer, colon cancer, lung cancer, melanoma, kidney cancer, pancreatic cancer, leukemia, thyroid cancer, and prostate cancer.
- 90 to 95 percent of cancer cases are due to lifestyle as well as environmental factors, and the rest of the 5 percent are due to genetics.
- More than 30 percent of cancer cases could be prevented, mainly by not using tobacco, having a healthy diet, being physically active, and preventing infections that may cause cancer.

I am a breast cancer survivor, but that's not why I first went on chia. I first tried chia a couple years ago after going through chemically-induced menopause brought on by radiation and chemotherapy. I just found that I wasn't as sharp as I used to be. I felt as if my brain was constantly in a fog, my memory was fading, and I was so scattered. I assumed these were symptoms of menopause. A friend told me about chia, which she was giving her son for ADHD symptoms. I tried it and after a couple weeks, felt more focused, more quick-witted.

As for the cancer, it is two years later and it hasn't returned. I'll continue to take chia to help keep my brain and cells healthy.

— ROBIN HANDLY, Brooklyn, NY

CARDIOVASCULAR CONDITIONS

Heart disease—also known as cardiovascular disease or CVD—affects one out of every four Americans each year (about 57 million people). It encompasses several related conditions of the heart, arteries, and veins, all of which supply oxygen to life-sustaining areas of the body such as the brain, the heart itself, and other vital organs. Here's an easy way to think about it: if an organ or tissue doesn't get the oxygen it needs, it will die.

Hypertension is a form of heart disease, as is stroke, arrhythmias (irregular heartbeats), angina (chronic chest pain), coronary artery diseases (atherosclerosis or clogged arteries, caused by a narrowing of the arteries or a buildup of cholesterol and other substances), and heart attacks.

Most cardiovascular diseases are caused by lifestyle choices—and thus can also be prevented and even treated with healthier lifestyle choices. Consuming chia daily is a lifestyle choice—and a good one, if you want to ward off, lessen, or help treat heart disease.

Very few formal studies have looked at chia's heart-health benefits, although this is changing. In a 2007 study from the University of Toronto, researchers fed 21 diabetics either a supplement made from chia or grains with a similar fiber content. After three months, blood pressure in patients taking chia dropped (10 points diastolic, 5 points systolic) while the grain group's blood pressure remained steady. Furthermore, researchers found that blood-clotting factors dropped 20 percent and levels of C-reactive protein, a marker of inflammation in heart disease, fell 30 percent.

Research at Oxford University, and at the University of Sydney, in Australia, and published in 2003 in the *European Journal of*

Nutrition, found a correlation between high flavenol intake and low heart disease mortality rates. Flavenols are antioxidants found in some plant foods, and are especially high in chia.

The March 2011 issue of *Journal of Nutritional Biochemistry* highlighted an Australian study from the University of Queensland, which found that the alpha-linolenic acid in chia seeds help reduce cardiac inflammation and fibrosis (thickening of the heart valves) in rats that ate a chia-enhanced diet for eight weeks.

It's tempting to list study after study, but suffice it to say that chia is chock-full of substances that can help protect your heart against cardiovascular disease. All you need are just two tablespoons a day.

HEART DISEASE FACTS

- Coronary heart disease is the most common type of cardiovascular disease (CVD).
- More than 50 percent of heart attack sufferers wait two hours or more before seeking help.
- Brain death from cardiac arrest can be experienced in just four minutes.
- A person with a family history of heart disease is ten times more likely to have cardiovascular disease.
- A diet high in fat and carbohydrates will increase the risk of blood clotting.
- About 47 percent of sudden cardiac deaths occur outside a hospital. This suggests that many people with heart disease don't act on early warning signs.
- Risk factors for a heart attack are high cholesterol, high blood pressure, sedentary lifestyle, obesity, poor diet, diabetes, high alcohol consumption, and smoking.
- Heart disease is the leading cause of death for both men and women.
- In 2010, heart disease cost the United States $316.4 billion. This total includes the cost of health care services, medications, and lost productivity.
- Every year about 785,000 Americans have a first heart attack. An additional 470,000 Americans who have already had one or more heart attacks have another attack.
- About 82 percent of people who die of coronary heart disease are 65 or older. At older ages, women who have heart attacks are more likely than men are to die from them within a few weeks.
- Smokers' risk of developing coronary heart disease is two to four times that of nonsmokers. People who smoke a pack of cigarettes a day have more than twice the risk of heart attack than people who've never smoked.
- Exposure to other people's smoke increases the risk of heart disease even for nonsmokers.

HEART DISEASE: OTHER WAYS TO HELP YOURSELF

Consuming chia regularly is a fantastic way to keep your cardiovascular system healthy. But there are plenty of other things you can do to ensure things run smoothly:

- Lower stress. While medical researchers don't know exactly how stress increases the risk of heart disease, they do know it contributes to poor cardiovascular health. When you are under stress, it is common to experience a rise in blood pressure, poor eating habits, and reliance on alcohol and cigarettes to self-soothe. Also, the stress hormones adrenaline and cortisol, which are released when you are stressed, can increase the risk of heart attack.

- Stop drinking. Over-drinking can raise the levels of fats (triglycerides) in the blood. Alcohol can also lead to high blood pressure, higher calorie intake (which can in turn contribute to obesity), and heart failure—or, in the case of binge drinking—a stroke. A few glasses of wine a week probably won't hurt you, but try to keep your weekly intake down to five servings or less.

- Cut out cigarettes. Chemicals in tobacco can damage your heart and blood vessels, leading to narrowing of the arteries. Called atherosclerosis, the condition hinders the passage of oxygen and can ultimately lead to a heart attack. The nicotine in cigarettes is also dangerous, making your heart work harder by narrowing your blood vessels and increasing your blood pressure. Furthermore, the carbon monoxide in cigarette smoke replaces some of the oxygen in your blood. This increases your blood pressure by forcing your heart to work harder to supply your body with enough oxygen.

- Get enough sleep. Poor sleep has been linked with high blood pressure, atherosclerosis, heart failure, heart attack and stroke, diabetes, and obesity. Though it's not understood exactly how lack of sleep and CVD are connected, researchers believe inflammation may be the culprit.

- Lose weight. Most people gain weight as they age, which is natural. However, being overweight forces your heart to work harder than it should; it also increases the chance you'll have high cholesterol and high blood pressure.

- Exercise. Physical activity helps you control your weight and can reduce your chances of developing other conditions that may put a strain on your heart, such as high blood pressure, high cholesterol, and diabetes. It also reduces stress, which may be a factor in heart disease.

- Eat a heart-healthy diet. When eating a heart-healthy diet, think farm, not factory. Whole, natural foods—vegetables especially—are at the core of a heart-supportive eating plan. The American Heart Association espouses "DASH," which stands for Dietary Approaches to Stop Hypertension. This includes eating plenty of plant foods, making sure that foods are low in cholesterol, fat, and salt, and going easy on animal products.

continues>

- Surround yourself with positive people. Several studies suggest that having a strong social network may help protect against heart disease. A study by the University of Minnesota in Minneapolis, looked at nearly 15,000 men and women between 1999 and 2002, and found that those who go to church and social clubs, and have a lot of friends and relatives, have significantly lower blood pressure and other heart disease risk factors than loners.
- Get a pet. A 10-year study of more than 4,435 Americans, aged 30 to 75, by researchers at the University of Minnesota's Stroke Institute in Minneapolis, found that owning a pet could reduce your risk of a heart attack by nearly one-third. It is believed that pet ownership helps people cope with, and overcome, daily stress.

My wife and children have been taking chia for a year. My wife began taking it when she started running marathons, and as her running partner, I see how much more endurance and strength she has—especially toward the end of a run. I also see how much faster my children's nails grow and that they seem more calm and focused when taking chia regularly. You'd think I would have jumped on the chia wagon with them, but I didn't begin taking it until I was diagnosed with hypertension. My blood pressure reading was 150 over 90. I came straight home from the doctor's office and pulled out the bag of chia, taking my first taste. I committed to taking 2 tablespoons every day. Now, three months later, my blood pressure reading is 120/80 and I hope to get it down even lower in the next few months.

—DANIEL KENNEDY, Costa Mesa, CA

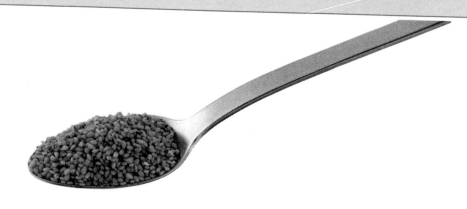

CHOLESTEROL

Cholesterol is on everyone's mind these days. Is yours high? Is it low? What is good cholesterol? What is bad cholesterol?

Before we get much further, let's talk about what cholesterol is. For you biochemistry buffs, cholesterol is a steroid alcohol produced by the liver. In fact, cholesterol is the most prominent steroid in the human body. This waxy substance helps the body manufacture hormones, vitamin D, and substances (such as bile), that help you digest foods. Your body makes all the cholesterol it needs.

However, bodies sometimes manufacture excess cholesterol. Or, they get additional cholesterol from animal foods. Because cholesterol cannot dissolve, your body may have more cholesterol than it can use. Trying to tidy itself up, the body shunts the unneeded cholesterol against artery walls, where it builds up, making arteries more and more narrow. Soon, oxygen-rich blood struggles to pass through these cluttered veins. (Just think of the hallways in your home. What would happen if you started stacking your unused stuff along the hallway walls. Soon, the hallways would be so cramped, you wouldn't be able to move through them.) The result is a number of cardiovascular diseases, including high blood pressure, stroke, and heart attacks.

Excess cholesterol can usually be managed with a few well-chosen lifestyle changes. The easiest is eating less animal foods, which contain cholesterol. Regular exercise boosts blood circulation, strengthens the heart muscle, and can help dislodge cholesterol buildup. Cutting out cigarettes and cutting down on alcohol (two things that also leads to cholesterol buildup) also helps.

Then there is chia, a wonder ingredient for lowering cholesterol levels. Though there have been no formal studies on the effects of chia on human cholesterol, studies in rats have shown that chia seed reduces blood fat and increases good cholesterol levels.

Furthermore, the alpha-linolenic acid in chia has been shown to reduce fat build up

My daughter was hounding me to eat chia to help lower my cholesterol but I thought she was crazy. Finally I said 'I'll show you—it won't work'. I started putting a tablespoon of chia in my orange juice every day and changed nothing else. In 60 days my cholesterol went down by 40 points. Now it is the lowest it has ever been at 150.
—PETER WIERCINSKI, submitted online to azchia.com

in arteries by lowering cholesterol levels. According to the American Heart Association, diets high in alpha-linolenic acid—the essential omega-3 fatty acid—have been associated with a 70 percent drop in coronary heart disease, compared with typical American diets that are low in this important omega-3 fatty acid.

Aim for two tablespoons of chia a day. If you are on medication, talk to your health care provider before consuming chia, just to be safe. However, there have been no known of complications or problems with chia.

> *Chia makes me feel great—full of energy and lowered my cholesterol significantly!*
> —DIANE SEARS,
> submitted online to azchia.com

GOOD CHOLESTEROL, BAD CHOLESTEROL

There are two types of cholesterol. One is called low-density lipoprotein. Think of this as "lousy cholesterol." The other type of cholesterol is called high-density lipoprotein. Think of this as good cholesterol. Whether it is lousy or good cholesterol, it cannot dissolve. Ideally, it hangs around the body only as long as it is needed to help create hormones and vitamins that assist with certain bodily processes. Once it's done what it is supposed to do, it heads to the liver, where it is passed from the body.

Lousy cholesterol, however, likes to hang out and party. It doesn't want to leave. It wants to stay and cause trouble. True, a few troublemakers in life are unavoidable. It's when you have too many that things get difficult. Enter good cholesterol. These conscientious workers do their jobs, swoop over, and strong-arm the LDL cholesterol to the liver, where they all leave the body together. If you don't have enough HDL cholesterol to help rid the body of troublemaking LDL cholesterol, you've got a problem—one that can be fixed with a combination of lifestyle interventions (diet and exercise) and possibly medication.

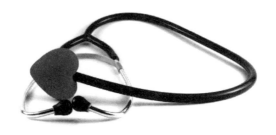

CHOLESTEROL FACTS

- Approximately one in every six adults—16.3 percent of the U.S. adult population—has high total cholesterol. The level defined as high total cholesterol is 240 mg/dL (milligrams per decilitre) and above.
- People with high total cholesterol have approximately twice the risk of heart disease as people with optimal levels. A desirable level is lower than 200 mg/dL.
- For adult Americans, the average level is about 200 mg/dL, which is borderline high risk.
- High blood cholesterol usually has no signs or symptoms. Thus, many people don't know that their cholesterol levels are too high.
- The American Heart Association recommends that daily dietary cholesterol intake not exceed 300 mg.
- Other names for high cholesterol are hypercholesterolemia and hyperlipidemia.
- More women than men have high cholesterol in the United States. The National Cholesterol Education Program recommends that all adults have their cholesterol levels checked once every five years.
- New Zealand has the highest per capita death rate from heart disease.
- Atherosclerosis, the clogging of arteries that can lead to heart attacks and strokes, can start before birth.
- One in five American teenagers has elevated cholesterol levels.
- Most of the cholesterol in your body is made in your liver, using saturated fat from your diet. Cholesterol also comes directly from some foods such as eggs, meats, and dairy products.

DIABETES

You've probably heard that diabetes is on the rise. You may even know that diabetes has something to do with blood sugar. But what, exactly is diabetes? And what causes it? Diabetes is considered a metabolism disorder, a glitch in the way our bodies use digested food for energy. You see, much of what we eat is broken down into a special type of fuel called glucose, a type of sugar found in the blood, and used by the body to fuel every bodily function.

The thing about glucose, however, is it cannot enter our cells alone. It needs to be escorted into cells by a special hormone called insulin.

Diabetes occurs when a person doesn't have enough insulin to escort the glucose into cells. This is called Type 1 diabetes. Or when a person consumes too much, creating more glucose than the body can handle. Or even, in some cases, when a body's cells simply ignore the insulin when it shows up with glucose. These are known as Type 2 diabetes. In all instances, the result is the same: too much glucose sitting around in the blood, unused, waiting to be utilized.

Like most illnesses, diabetes has signs. Some of the most obvious are frequent urination (when there is too much glucose—sugar—in your blood you will urinate more often in order to dilute it), urgent thirst, intense hunger, weight gain (or, in some instances, unusual weight loss), increased fatigue, irritability, blurred vision, cuts and bruises that don't heal well, an increase in skin infections, yeast infections, itchy skin, swollen gums, frequent gum infections, sexual dysfunction in men, and numbness or tingling in hands and feet.

Fortunately, all types of diabetes are treatable: Type 1, mainly by injectable insulin, plus some dietary and exercise adherence; Type 2, with exercise and a special diet, though in more severe cases insulin injections may also be required.

Chia can help both types of diabetes by slowing the rate of carbohydrates' conversion into sugar, thus helping to maintain healthy blood sugar levels. Chia gel surrounds carbohydrates during digestion, slowing their release into the blood stream and helping to moderate blood sugar levels. In a 2007 study

performed at the St. Michael's Hospital in Toronto and reported in *Diabetes Care* magazine, 20 subjects with Type 2 diabetes were given 37 grams of chia seed a day (that's roughly three tablespoons) for 12 weeks. Not only did the chia help control blood sugar, it reduced the subject's risk markers for cardiovascular disease by lowering blood pressure, and reducing harmful LDL cholesterol and triglycerides, while increasing beneficial HDL cholesterol.

Further, a five-month study at the University of Litoral in Santa Fe, Argentina, found that rats that ate a high-sugar diet were less likely to suffer from insulin resistance when they consumed daily chia than control rats that were not given chia.

THE IMPORTANCE OF MANAGING DIABETES.

If you think you have diabetes, it's important to see a medical professional and create a treatment plan—hopefully one that includes chia! If diabetes is not adequately controlled you run the risk of developing complications, including erectile dysfunction, hypoglycemia, ketoacidosis, cardiovascular disease, retinal damage, chronic kidney failure, nerve damage, poor healing of wounds, gangrene on the feet, which may lead to amputation, and ultimately coma.

DIGESTIVE HEALTH

Irritable bowel syndrome, diverticulitis, constipation, and other digestive ills—the symptoms differ—are caused by one thing: a poorly-functioning large intestine, usually caused by lack of fiber. These common ills are thought to affect more than one-third of adults under the age of 45, half of Americans between the ages of 46 and 80, and two-thirds of Americans over the age of 80. That's a lot of people! Not only do digestive conditions make individuals feel miserable, they compromise nutrient absorption, contribute to fatigue and sluggishness, and in severe cases, contribute to colorectal cancer.

That's because when partially digested food spends a lot of time in the large intestine, bile acid gets re-absorbed, bad bacteria grows unchecked and good bacteria is smothered, harmful toxins build-up in a crowded colon and can even be absorbed by the body.

While chia has not been researched specifically for digestive issues, fiber has. Several studies in the U.S. and the European Union

PSYLLIUM VS. CHIA

If you've been taking psyllium to get your daily dose of insoluble fiber, here's good news: You can go with chia and get not only fiber, but omega-3, antioxidants, and protein. To obtain the same amount of soluble fiber as found in a gram of psyllium, however, you need to consume approximately 20 grams of chia, which will bring to about 7.18 grams of insoluble fiber, and 1.07 grams of soluble fiber to boot.

have found that 20 to 35 grams of fiber a day keeps digestion regular and lowers risk of colorectal cancer. (The average American adult gets less than 15 grams daily.) Chia contains about 5 grams of fiber per tablespoon. Three tablespoons per day are enough to improve digestive health and comfort.

And yet the fiber in chia definitely aids in keeping the large intestine moving things along efficiently and easily. But roughage isn't the only thing at work. Chia, which is highly hydrophilic, brings moisture to the large intestine. As it moves through the colon, it "irrigates" the intestine, keeping the contents moist and malleable.

I've been using 1 tablespoon of milled chia in 8 oz of water daily and it's helped keep my digestion regular.

—KATHLEEN KORTH,
submitted online to azchia.com

DRINK YOUR WATER!

Most Americans don't drink enough water, which can lead to constipation. After all, the body needs water to keep waste products moving efficiently through and out. Because chia swells 9 to 12 times its size in the stomach, it is especially important to get enough liquid to help the body utilize chia. Aim for one 8-ounce glass of water or other liquid for each tablespoon of chia you consume.

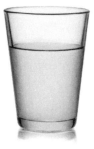

FATIGUE

Chia had many uses among the Aztecs, who were the first to document its use. One of the most important ways they used the seed was as an energy booster and endurance aid. Story after story has emerged from the Aztec codices (see page 9) on how their warriors, traveling messengers, and athletes sustained themselves on a daily spoonful of chia and a measure of water. In Christopher McDougall's book, *Born to Run*, he talks to the possible descendants of the Aztecs, native people living in Mexico's Copper Canyon. These super athletes are famous for their 100-mile (or longer) runs, fueled by nothing more than chia seed and water.

How does chia boost endurance? A few ways, probably. Chia is hydrophilic, meaning it helps the body retain moisture, guarding it against energy-sapping dehydration, as well as protecting joints from the wear and tear of intense physical activity.

The seed's high nutrient profile also helps sustain energy. With a wide range of protein, vitamins, minerals, amino acids, fatty acid, and antioxidants, chia delivers the nutrition body systems need to run efficiently at peak performance, as well as the omega-3 fatty acid needed to quickly repair itself.

I have taken chia over 3 months now and can tell you that it provides me with stable energy, appetite suppression, and better digestion. The amount of Omega-3 is so good for my clarity and focus daily as a business coach and mentor.

—JACOB ROIG,
submitted online to azchia.com

INFLAMMATORY CONDITIONS

Inflammation is a hot word in health circles these days, and with good reason. Recent research has found that inflammation at the root of a host of illnesses, and some scientists theorize that inflammation is the very thing that causes aging.

Heart disease, arthritis, acne, asthma, allergies, food sensitivities and intolerances, pelvic inflammatory disease, inflammatory bowel disease, and autoimmune system diseases are just a few examples of inflammatory disease. They occur when some of the body's cells (different conditions involve different cells) are irritated by something—maybe bacteria, a virus, a chemical, or even dramatic change in temperature. The affected cells react by swelling. Blood floods the area, trying to send healing oxygen to the aggrieved cells. Plasma leaks into the area, making it swell further. All the activity may raise the temperature of the cells. In some cases, the swelling spreads to affect other parts of the body.

Soon the immune system is working overtime, either adding to the cells' angry response or trying to calm them down. This large expenditure of energy takes the body's energy away from its normal body systems, maintenance, and other functions. The result is fatigue, immune system dysfunction, in some cases a chronic condition, and even cancer in other cases.

Chia can help. Generous amounts of antioxidants help strengthen the immune system and prevent cells from over-reacting in the first place. The high levels of omega-3 fatty acid in chia help decrease inflammation, normalizing the affected area.

IMMUNE SYSTEM FUNCTION

Any time you get a cold, a flu, or a virus, you can blame your immune system. This fascinating body system is in charge of keeping out foreign invaders—from parasites and bacteria to toxins and microbes—that may make you sick. It's also in charge of getting you well, should an invader have snuck in and wrought havoc on your health. If the virus or bacteria is able to reproduce and start causing problems, your immune system is in charge of eliminating it. The immune system also has several other important jobs. For example, your immune system can detect cancer in early stages and eliminate it in many cases.

Comprised of the thymus, spleen, lymph system, bone marrow, white blood cells, antibodies, and hormones, this complex system responds exquisitely to antioxidants—something chia has in generous amounts. Antioxidants strengthen the immune system, allowing it to protect you and battle invaders even more quickly and aggressively. The alpha-linolenic acid in chia also fortifies the immune system.

> *I had terrible bursitis, which I chalked up to age and a lifelong love of tennis. Last year I began taking one tablespoon of chia a day to help my nails grow longer. I know, vanity! But an interesting thing happened. My bursitis lessened. I upped my dose to 3 tablespoons a day and the pain completely left. I am chia's biggest fan!*
> —LORNA SEHR,
> Minneapolis, MN

IMMUNE SYSTEM FACTS

- The skin is a barrier that stops many germs from entering the body.
- The thymus is a gland in the chest, which turns ordinary white blood cells into special T-cells that fight harmful microbes.
- Some scientists believe that excess sugar decreases your body's immunity.
- Mucus lines your airways and lungs to protect them from smoke particles, as well as from germs. Your airways may fill up with mucus when you have a cold, as your body tries to minimize the invasion of airborne germs.
- The adenoids in the nose are one of the body's defense centers, releasing cells to fight infections.
- If you get a throat infection, the tonsils release cells to fight it.
- Did you know gum disease weakens the immune system? Flossing and brushing daily are easy ways to increase immune system function.
- Lymph glands in your groin often swell up as the body fights an infection.
- Sebaceous glands in the skin secrete an oil that is poisonous to many bacteria.
- Studies have shown that sleep, sex, laughter, calming music, and moderate exercise help fortify the immune system.
- Itching, sneezing, coughing, and vomiting are your body's most common ways of ousting unwelcome invaders.
- Small particles that get trapped in the mucous lining of your airways are pushed out by tiny hairs called cilia.
- Certain white blood cells are cytotoxic, which means that they are poisonous to invaders.
- The spleen not only destroys worn-out red blood cells, it also helps make antibodies and phagocytes.
- White blood cells called phagocytes are drawn to the site of an infection whenever there is inflammation. These cells swallow up invaders and then use an enzyme to dissolve them.

My daughter began taking chia to help calm and focus her. What I noticed, however, is that as we approached cold and flu season, she never got sick. I used to have to keep her home at least twice a year for various colds, but since starting a tablespoon of chia each day, she hasn't had a single sick day.

—TRACI WALKER, Reno, NV

BRAIN & NERVOUS SYSTEM HEALTH

The nervous system is in charge of keeping you calm, cool, and collected. But sometimes the nervous system doesn't work as well as it should. The result is depression, ADHD, anxiety, stress, and a host of other mood and behavior disorders.

Medication is an option for those suffering from severe nervous system conditions. But for many people, regular exercise, sleep, and an upgrade in nutrients is enough to put them back on course. Chia is a great help under these circumstances. Research has shown that deficiencies in omega-3 fatty acids are contributing factors in many mood disorders, depression among them. One of the most-cited studies is an eight-week trial conducted in 2010 at McGill University in Montreal. It found that omega-3 supplements helped about half the patients with major depression.

Indeed, the omega-3 fatty acids in chia have been shown by other studies, as well, to nourish the brain and help create a sense of calm and focus. Chia's minerals and B-vitamins also lend a sense of calm focus while helping the nervous system to work more efficiently. Tryptophan, also found in chia, is an amino acid that helps the brain create serotonin and melatonin, two feel-good neurotransmitters.

I didn't begin taking chia for anxiety, but found it to be a wonderful help. I started to take it because my running coach suggested it. I noticed a big difference in my knees and hips after longer runs. I also noticed I was less reactive to stress at work and in my marriage. It gave me a kind of 'go with the flow' outlook that other people have commented on. My nails look great, too!
—MELINDA KOONS, Chicago, IL

I began to give chia seed to my eight-year-old standard poodle mix, who had come down with a flaky, itchy skin condition as he aged. My vet said the omega-3s in chia would help heal his skin and give him a nicer coat. She was right. But what we didn't expect was to see a softening of his disposition. He had always been a high-strung, slightly nervous dog, but about three weeks into the chia, we noticed that things he once reacted to didn't seem to bother him as much. He's been a much more pleasant dog—to look at, and to be around.
—BOB DOOLEY, Albany, NY

SKIN, NAILS, AND HAIR HEALTH

Skin is our largest organ—and one of our most visible markers of health. Skin is our greatest detoxifying organ, helping to release harmful substances from the body. It's also an important member of the immune system, working to keep pathogens and other invaders out.

When we're healthy, our skin is smooth, clear, and bright. When something is off—maybe we're not metabolizing nutrients the way we should, aren't getting enough sleep, or are suffering from some kind of illness—our skin gets oily, flaky, spotty, bumpy, sallow, splotchy. In other words, our skin doesn't look good.

Our fingernails, toenails, hair, eyebrows and eyelashes are appendages of the skin, meaning that whatever nourishes the skin, nourishes them. One of the nutrients that skin absolutely loves, is omega-3 fatty acids. Chia is full of them, in the form of alpha-linolenic acid, which improves skin by reducing any inflammation that can be causing spots, bumps, or acne. Chia's hydrophilic qualities draw moisture to the skin and hair, making them soft and supple. Chia's minerals harden nails and encourage hair and skin cell growth. At the same time, chia's high volume of antioxidants protect skin and its appendages from the ravages of bacteria, fungi, viruses, parasites, and environmental toxins, all of which can change the way skin looks and grows.

I had been eating chia for some time, but felt I could increase my intake easily by adding chia to my morning milk. It was not long until I noticed my hair was shinier and more easily managed. In fact my hair stylist made a comment on a recent visit that she noticed my hair was shinier and healthier.
—PATRICIA WIERCINSKI,
submitted online to azchia.com

HOW TO USE CHIA FOR BETTER SKIN

Whether you've got acne or wrinkles, chia can help your skin look better. The easiest way to tap into the looks-enhancing power of chia is simply by eating it. Try one or two tablespoons a day to start. If you've battling a stubborn skin condition, try three tablespoons a day. Of course, chia also can do wonders when placed on the skin. Opt for chia oil, or make your own chia skincare products (see pages 119–122 for more information).

Chia has been a tremendous help in keeping my skin inflammation under control. It is a great relief to use an all-natural food that works effectively, every day, eliminating the need for prescription steroid creams.
—LAUREN ROSEMOND,
submitted online to azchia.com

I have been using chia for about a year now. What a difference. I am a lot more calm. I can sleep. My cholesterol and blood pressure are great! My hair and nails are growing stronger and faster. I would recommend this to anyone, especially if you are starting menopause.
—MAUREEN SILVA,
submitted online to azchia.com

FREQUENTLY ASKED QUESTIONS

When you have an ingredient as powerful—and with as many wide-ranging benefits—as chia, there are bound to be questions. Here are some of the questions we see over and over again about this beneficial food.

NUTRIENTS AND BENEFITS

Q. Does chia have essential fatty acids?

A. Chia seed is the highest known plant source of omega-3 fatty acids. Two tablespoons of chia seed offers 5 grams of omega-3 fatty acids.

Q. What is an essential fatty acid?

A. Essential fatty acids are so called because they cannot be synthesized in the body; it is therefore essential to obtain them from foods. Omega-6 and omega-3 are the essential fatty acids for humans and other animals. They are precursors of powerful hormones that affect many biological processes; they help maintain healthy skin, and are involved in cholesterol metabolism.

Q. Is one omega-3 fatty acid better than another?

A. The only one that is essential is ALA (alpha-linolenic acid), the type of omega-3 found in chia. DHA and EPA, which come from marine sources, are not essential omega-3 fatty acids, since they can be synthe-sized by the body (converted from ALA).

Q. What is the appropriate omega-6 to omega-3 ratio?

A. The ideal ratio is from 1:1 to 3:1. During our evolutionary period, humans ate an omega-6/omega-3 ratio of 1:1. Modern diets are very rich in omega-6, derived primarily from vegetable and animal fats. Typically, today's diets provide ratios that are greater than 15:1 omega-6 to omega-3. This imbalance increases the risk of coronary heart disease and also heightens the body's natural inflammatory processes.

Q. How do omega-6 and omega-3 fatty acids compare?

A. In general, omega-3's are anti-inflammatory, whereas omega-6's are just the opposite—they promote inflammation.

Q. What are the other sources of omega-3 fatty acid?

A. In general, omega-3 is present in fatty, wild sea fish and in green vegetables. Most oil crops have very little of this fatty acid. Sea fish have omega-3 only if they are wild and get if from a marine source. Farm-raised sea fish must be fed omega-3 supplements in order to provide omega-3.

Q. Can I get too much of the omega-3 fatty acids in chia?
A. The omega-3 fatty acid in chia is called alpha-linolenic acid, or ALA. You can eat up to a cup of chia a day and your body is going to convert just the amount of ALA your body needs. That need varies from person to person, so your body is going to convert ALA differently than mine. What your body doesn't use will be excreted.

Q. Can I lose weight eating chia?
A. Chia has high amounts of fiber (both soluble and insoluble), which is low in calories. Two tablespoons will give you 8.25 grams of fiber. Furthermore, since chia is highly hydrophilic (it absorbs water), it expands in the stomach, giving you a pleasant feeling of satiety or fullness—if you feel full, you'll be less likely to overeat.

Q. What is the difference between soluble and insoluble fiber?
A. Soluble fiber is "swellable" in water. When it's mixed with liquid, soluble forms a gel-like substance and swells. It is great for moderating blood glucose levels and lowering cholesterol. Soluble fiber is found in peas, beans, lentils, oatmeal, and the pectin of fruit.

Insoluble fiber does not swell or dissolve in water and passes through the digestive system in much the same way it entered the system. Insoluble fiber is great for intestinal health, helps with constipation, hemorrhoids, and colorectal cancer.

Q. What minerals does chia have?
A. Boron, calcium, copper, iodine, iron, magnesium, manganese, molybdenum, phosphorus, potassium, silicon, sodium, strontium, sulfur, and zinc. It also has amylose (a slow-burning starch helpful in treating hypoglycemia) and plenty of electrolytes.

Q. What vitamins does chia have?
A. The main vitamins are: A, B1 (Thiamin), B2 (Riboflavin), C (ascorbic acid), E, choline, and Folate (folic acid). Chia also contains vitamins B3, B5, B6, B15, B17, D, K, inositol, and PABA.

Q. What else does chia contain?
A. Linoleic acid, antioxidants, including chlorogenic and caffeic acids, myricetin, quercetin, and kaempferol flavonol, chlorogenic acid, caffeic acid, flavonol glycosides, mucin, fiber, and 18 of the 22 amino acids, including all nine essential amino acids:

isoleucine, leucine, lysine, methionine, phenylalanine, threonine, tryptophan, valine, and histadine.

Q. Is chia good for persons with arthritis?
A. Chia is very good for people with arthritis or any type of joint pain, because it is high in omega-3 fatty acid and antioxidants, which are powerful anti-inflammatory agents.

Q. Can chia be eaten by people who have celiac disease or are gluten intolerant?
A. Chia seed is gluten-free and can be eaten by people suffering from celiac disease.

Q. Could chia cause problems in people with diverticulitis?
A. In general, the fiber in chia protects the intestine walls and improves the process of digestion. Grinding chia in a coffee mill or using milled chia is an option since chia in this form has a much smaller particle size, which some people find easier to process. People with specific digestive problems should consult their doctors about the best form to use.

Q. Is it the fiber in chia that helps with conditions like diverticulitis and IBS?
A. Yes, the fiber in chia definitely aids in keeping the large intestine moving things along efficiently and easily, but roughage isn't the only thing at work. Chia, which is highly hydrophilic, brings moisture to the large intestine. As it moves through the colon, it "irrigates" the intestine, keeping the contents moist and malleable.

Q. I have been eating psyllium for fiber. Can I eat chia instead?
A. Definitely. The advantage with chia is that in addition to the fiber, you also get omega-3, antioxidants, and protein. To obtain the same amount of fiber as found in a gram of psyllium, however, you need to consume approximately two grams of chia. With a recommended daily amount of 15 or more grams of chia (a little over a tablespoon), you would get as much fiber as what is generally recommended for daily consumption of psyllium.

Q. My personal trainer said I should have chia daily between weight lifting workouts. Why?
A. Chia is believed to decrease recovery time and fatigue in cardiovascular workouts by encouraging muscle tissue repair.

Q. I've heard chia is great for diabetics. Why?

A. Chia seeds slow the conversion rate of carbohydrates into sugar, thus helping to maintain healthy blood-sugar levels. Chia gel surrounds carbohydrates during digestion, according to Penni Shelton, in her book *Raw Food Cleanse*, slowing the release of carbohydrates into the blood stream and helping to moderate blood sugar levels.

Q. I'm a long-distance runner. What can chia do for me?

A. Chia is hydrophilic and can absorb between 9 and 12 times its weight in water. This means that chia increases body hydration, which is especially beneficial for athletes who need to remain hydrated during long races and endurance activities.

Q. What happens after I've swallowed chia?

A. When chia reaches the digestive liquids of your stomach, it swells and forms a gel. This gel slows down the rate at which digestive enzymes turn carbohydrates into sugar. This makes chia fantastic for diabetics, people with blood sugar irregularities, and for those who experience cravings related to glucose levels.

Q. I understand I should drink plenty of liquids when eating chia. Why?

A. Since chia absorbs a lot of liquid, it can lead to stomach cramps. Hence the need to consume sufficient liquid when consuming chia.

Q. I'm looking for a way to get more easily assimilated minerals into my diet. Can chia help?

A. Yes! Chia contains an impressive dose of several minerals, including boron to help the body assimilate calcium. In addition, chia contains: more than five times the amount of calcium in one serving of milk; 15 times more magnesium than broccoli; two times more potassium than a banana; and three times more iron than spinach.

Q. I heard Dr. Oz say that chia helps promote sound sleep. How?

A. Chia is rich in tryptophan, the amino acid that raises the level of natural sleep aids, melatonin and serotonin, in the body. Two ounces of chia has twice the amount of tryptophan as a serving of turkey. Try taking chia two or three hours before bedtime–or find a way to add chia to your evening meal.

Q. I've heard chia can make my nails healthier and grow faster. Is it true?

A. Chia is rich in omega-3, as well as calcium,

boron, and many antioxidants that help create healthy, moist, disease-free skin. Nails and hair are appendages of the skin, which means that anything that makes the skin healthier will also make nails and hair healthier. Incidentally, one thing I noticed about chia is that it helped me complete ultra-distant runs. The second thing I noticed was how strong and healthy my nails looked. So yes, chia is very beneficial to nails.

Q. Can chia seed be used on the skin?

A. Yes, when mixed with water into a gel, chia is very moisturizing and refreshing when applied to the skin. Some indigenous people even used chia gel as a poultice to prevent infection and promote healing in wounds.

Q. Can I take chia oil capsules?

A. Yes, chia oil capsules provide generous amounts of omega-3 fatty acids, but you'd be missing out on the fiber and protein that are available in chia seed. At press time, there have been no clinical trials studying the nutritional profile and isolated benefits of chia oil.

Q. Can I use chia oil on my skin?

A. Yes. A Korean study published in the May 2010 issue of *Annals of Dermatology* reported that chia gel was effective in treating eczema, pruritus, and other itchy skin conditions.

CHIA VERSUS FLAX

Q. Does chia need to be ground, like flax, in order to digest it and benefit from its high omega-3 content?

A. The way I like to explain the difference is as follows: Mother Nature prevents the omega-3 in flaxseed from going rancid by a hard seed coat. In the case of chia, the omega-3 content is protected by the natural antioxidants in the seed.

What this means for you is that if you want to get the benefits of omega-3 from flaxseed, you need to grind, cook, sprout, or somehow open the seed so that the digestive process can be effective. If you do not do this, the seeds will just pass through your body. This is not the case with chia: You can eat the whole seed, and you will get essentially all of the benefits of the omega-3 as well as the other components in this very special food.

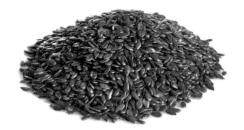

Q. I actually prefer to grind my chia. Does it go rancid as quickly as flax?

A. No. In fact, the second advantage which chia has over flax seed is that if you do like to eat milled (ground) chia, you can prepare it, leave it on your countertop, and it will not go rancid. This is very different from flax seed, which should be kept in the refrigerator and ground fresh every day. Why is this the case? Again, this advantage comes from the natural antioxidants in chia seeds, which prevent rancidity.

Q. What is the history of flaxseed use and chia, are there differences?
A. Chia has long been used as a food in Central America, not only for humans but for animals as well. On the other hand, flaxseed and flax do not have a long history as a food. Historically, flax has more commonly been used for fiber (linen), paper products, and oil for paints, preservatives, etc. For example, where do the words linoleum and linseed oil come from? They are derived from the word lino, which is the word used for flaxseed in other countries.

Q. Does chia contain lignans like flax does?
A. No, and this is a good thing. Lignan is a class of phytoestrogen with antioxidant activity. It is found in some plant foods, though flax is the highest source. It is the lignans in flax that contribute to flax's estrogenic activity, which can affect fertility and may contribute to estrogen-dominant cancers.

Q. I've heard my vegan friends say that chia makes a better egg substitute in homemade baked goods than flax does. How does that work?
A. When mixed with water into a gel, chia helps add moisture, elasticity, and cohesiveness to baked goods. Try mixing two tablespoons of ground chia or chia seed, with two tablespoons of water for each egg needed. Allow the mixture to sit for a few minutes until it has gelled. Add it to your recipe, just as you would an egg.

Q. How can I use chia to replace an egg white?
A. To replace one medium or large egg white, use 1 teaspoon milled chia with ⅛ cup water. There is one caveat, however: Chia cannot be whipped into stiff peaks like egg whites, so use real eggs for making meringue.

CONSUMING & STORING CHIA
Q. What does chia taste like?
A. Chia doesn't really have a distinct flavor. I'd say the flavor is a bit nutty and slightly malty, but, for me, the flavor is so mild that it's more about the crunch than the taste.

Q. How can I eat chia?
A. Chia seeds can be consumed directly and do not need to be ground. Most people mix them with foods such as yogurt, juices, broths, salads, omelets, cereals, etc. In addi-

tion, chia can be mixed (ground or whole) with flour and used for making breads, muffins, desserts, pizza, etc. Some people even put it on their ice cream as a nutty topping!

Q. How much chia should I eat each day?

A. There is no definitive answer to this question. Since chia is a food, there really is no limit to how much you can eat. One of the main reasons a person eats chia is to obtain omega-3. The obvious question is how much chia will give you a sufficient amount of omega-3. The 2010 Dietary Guidelines for Americans states that an adequate intake of alpha-linolenic acid (the form of omega-3 in chia), ranges between 1.1 and 1.6 grams/day for adults. Since 12 to 18 grams (2 to 3 teaspoons) of chia contain between 2.5 and 3.6 grams of alpha linoleic acid, this is more than a sufficient amount to meet this recommendation.

Q. I am a vegan. Should I eat chia?

A. A recent study showed that vegetarians, and vegans in particular, typically have low levels of omega-3 fatty acids in their plasma. This can lead to serious coronary problems. Hence it is especially important for these groups of individuals to increase their omega-3 consumption. Chia is the highest plant source of omega-3, making it an excellent choice to meet this need.

Q. Which chia product is easiest to eat on

a daily basis, whole or milled?

A. Whether you choose to eat chia, whole or milled, is truly a personal preference and depends on the food you are adding it to. Do you like the crunchy aspect of the whole seed or not? Again, it's a personal choice.

Q. Is it necessary to grind the seed?

A. Chia seeds do not need to be ground for absorption, unlike flax, which must be ground before eating it.

Q. There is so-called "ground" chia available. What does this refer to?

A. Grinding as it applies to wheat, for example, cannot be used to break open chia seed. This is due to the high oil content of the seed, and grinding it would essentially turn the seed into a paste. Such a process would also heat the seed and lead to oxidation, resulting in decreased oil quality and a rancid flavor and smell. Several processing methods can be used to open chia seeds— and all of them use similar techniques. These processes are similar to those that are used to grind flaxseed, none of which are patented as far as I am aware. Personally, I prefer to use the term "milled" rather than ground.

Q. Can I grind—or mill—chia at home?

A. Yes, you can mill chia at home. Simply whir the chia seeds for a few seconds in a coffee grinder. Just be careful not to overdo it. Thanks to chia's high oil content, you can be left with chia butter in no time.

Q. Although chia is known to contain about 20 percent protein, is it a high-quality protein?

A. Yes it is. Chia has been given an amino acid score of 115. Any amino acid score over 100 indicates it is a complete or high-quality protein.

Q. Should chia seeds be washed?

A. Chia seeds do not need to be washed. Furthermore, if chia seeds are placed in water, their high level of soluble fiber will absorb moisture (up to 9 times their weight) and form a gel.

Q. Is it necessary to soak the seed?

A. Chia seeds do not need to be soaked, although some people like to make a gel, which is the soluble fiber coming from the seed, by placing the seed in water, but this is not necessary. If you make a gel, it should be refrigerated, and will keep for about a week.

Q. I drink a tablespoon of chia each morning in a glass of water. I love how energetic I feel, but I hate cleaning the chia seeds off the glass—they really stick. Help!

A. They are sticky, aren't they? What I do is add a drop of dish soap, fill the glass with cold water, and get a bottle brush out. The stuck seeds wash away pretty easily.

Q. How exactly, does chia swell when wet?

A. The outside of the chia seed is covered in tiny micro-fibers. When the seed is wet, these nearly-invisible tiny fibers stand on end and begin trapping liquid. This property is so amazing, the seed can hold nine times its weight in water! This action causes a bead of gel to form around the seed.

Q. Is it better to eat the seed or the chia oil capsules?

A. It depends on what you want to achieve. People who are interested in a rich source of omega-3, but also want a good source of fiber, protein, minerals, and vitamins prefer to eat the seed. If the only interest is increasing omega-3 in the diet, then the oil capsules will provide an excellent source. In terms of value, the seed is a much better option.

Q. What is chia fresca?

A. This is a beverage made by adding chia, lime juice, and a bit of sugar to water. It is consumed in some parts of Mexico, where it is considered a refreshing summer drink.

Q. How should chia seeds be stored?
A. Whole chia seeds will stay in good condition at room temperature for several years. There is no need to keep the seeds in the refrigerator, whether it's kept in sealed bags or not. The seed's natural antioxidants provide this stability. Milled chia seeds can be left on the countertop for approximately a year. Storing chia in a closed container will help extend its shelf life.

Q. How long can I keep chia sitting around?
A. I like to say two years just to ensure that you have the freshest tasting chia, but it will stay fresh for four or five years with no problem.

Q. Do I have to consume a lot of chia in order for it to be effective?
A. No. In 1891, for instance, botanist Edward Palmer explored Mexico, consuming one teaspoon of chia per 24 hours of foot travel. This amount was sufficient to sustain him.

Q. We love lightly toasting chia seeds in a pan, will this degrade the omega-3 content?
A. Just like baking, there is no evidence that the omega-3 content will be reduced in terms of quantity or quality. Temperature is the key aspect here. For example you should not fry the seeds since this could lead to degradation, however baking or lightly toasting chia should not cause a problem.

Q. Dr. Coates, what's your favorite way to eat chia?
A. In a peanut butter sandwich, made with crunchy peanut butter. I love crunch, and between the crunch of the peanuts and the crunch of the chia, I am in heaven. When I run, however, I fill film canisters with chia, then tuck the canisters into my running belt. Whenever I need extra energy, I open a container, swallow half the contents, and then wash the chia down with a swallow or two of water.

Q. My friend told me that chia must be soaked before eating in order to be digestible. Is this true?
A. No. Soaking chia does soften the seed somewhat and give it a gel-like consistency. This may be easier for some people to consume. But dry and milled chia are equally nutritious and digestible.

CHIA & SAFETY

Q. Is chia safe?

A. Chia has been consumed by humans for thousands of years. It was one of the main foods of the Aztecs and Mayans. The FDA has stated that chia is a food, rather than a supplement, and can be consumed without restrictions.

Q. Is chia seed a Genetically Modified Organism (GMO)?

A. No.

Q. Is chia seed organic? Are there insecticides or fungicides used?

A. There is certified organic chia seed. However, non-organic production can be considered environmentally friendly because the soil fertility is maintained, due to crop rotation and other conservation practices, and weed control is mechanical, instead of chemical. In fact, chemical pest control is not needed, since the plant is a member of the mint family. As such, insects never bother it, since the stem and leaves have essential oils that repel damaging insects.

Furthermore, spraying chia plants with insecticide would be counterproductive, since chia plants need insects for pollination. No fungicides are used, nor are any biological controls carried out during its production, cleaning, or processing.

Q. Is the chia oil in capsules expelled from seeds with chemicals?

A. To obtain chia oil, which is used in nutrient supplements, chia seed is generally cold pressed and no chemicals are added. Another system that is used to extract the oil is using high-pressure carbon dioxide, or other inert gases, to force out the oil. Again, no chemicals are added.

Q. Is chia oil stable, does it oxidize?

A. As with any omega-3 oil, oxidation is a problem. In some cases, stabilizers are added to the oil to keep it fresh longer. In general, however, either encapsulation or storing in a dark, sealed container, under refrigeration, will keep the oil fresh for a reasonable period of time.

Q. I thought you said chia had antioxidants, which keep it from going rancid?

A. This is true, however when the oil is extracted, the antioxidants do not pass into the oil.

Q. I have seen people selling chia flour, what is this?

A. Typically this refers to the press cake (what is left after most of the oil has been pressed out) which has been ground. This has a very low omega-3 content, but is higher in fiber and protein than the seed itself.

Q. I have heard that because chia contains omega-3 fatty acids, it can thin the blood, lower blood pressure to a dangerous level, and promote increased bleeding.
A. Studies have shown that DHA in particular, and EPA to a lesser extent, can lower blood pressure. These long chain forms of omega-3 fatty acids come from fish or algae oils. Chia contains the short chain form of omega-3, ALA (alpha-linolenic acid). There have been no reports that the ALA form of omega-3 fatty acids in chia causes such problems.

Q. Have any health issues arisen when consuming chia?
A. Limited trials have not found any allergic reactions to chia, even in nut-sensitive individuals. Chia is gluten-free, so individuals suffering from celiac disease can safely consume chia. Also, individuals with diabetes should have no issues consuming chia—in fact, the soluble fiber in chia appears to reduce glycemic spikes.

Q. Can I eat too much chia?
A. Not really. If you eat more than your body can handle, you may find yourself feeling a bit bloated, or you may experience mild diarrhoea, though this is rare.

Q. Is it possible to be allergic to chia?
A. It is very rare, but the possibility does exist. A reaction can be mild, such as a smattering of hives, or it can be a more severe anaphylactic reaction that requires an emergency room visit. Those most likely to have a reaction to chia are individuals who are allergic to sesame or mustard seed, or to other members of the salvia family, such as sage.

Q. I'm on medication. Can I take chia?
A. It depends on the medication. Because chia can delay stomach emptying, it can affect how medication is metabolized. Your best bet is to talk with your healthcare provider before taking chia.

Q. Does chia cause stomach cramps?
A. In some cases, stomach cramps have been reported, but these are due to a natural body reaction. This happens if a substantial amount of chia is eaten, and insufficient fluids are consumed with it. The cramping is caused because chia absorbs liquid from the stomach, placing it in a stressful state. The solution is to drink more liquid when consuming chia, or reduce the amount of chia consumed.

Q. I have heard chia causes diarrhea, is this true?
A. Some individuals have experienced diarrhea, but this has generally been reported with individuals who are on a low-fiber diet, and then suddenly increase the amount of

fiber consumed. This problem can easily be avoided: simply introduce chia to your diet slowly.

Q. Someone told me that chia is addictive. Is this true?
A. I know of no addiction to chia.

Q. Is chia good for pregnant women? I read on one website that chia thins the blood. If a pregnant woman has an emergency C-section, couldn't she bleed to death?
A. There is no evidence that I know of that chia thins the blood. Again one must be careful of what you read online; anyone can post information, whether it is correct, researched, made up, factual, false, or whatever. All patients should share their concerns with their doctors.

Q. Is chia FDA approved?
A. Chia seed is considered to be a safe food by the U.S. Food and Drug Administration (FDA). So yes, chia is FDA approved.

Q. Does chia contribute to prostate cancer? I read this somewhere.
A. In 2004, The Wageningen Centre for Food Science in the Netherlands published a small study indicating that chia could increase a man's risk of prostate cancer. More and larger studies, however, have shown that the high levels of antioxidants and fiber like those found in chia actually *prevent* prostate cancer. If you are at risk for or currently have prostate cancer, examine the research on chia and discuss it with your healthcare provider.

Q. Does chia lower blood pressure? Could chia help lower my hypertension?
A. It could. St. Michael's Hospital in Toronto found that chia seeds have the potential to drastically lower diastolic blood pressure. This is an enormous benefit for people who have high blood pressure. However, if you have low blood pressure, you should discuss chia with your healthcare provider before using it.

Q. My doctor recommends not eating chia, why?
A. Unfortunately, many doctors are totally unaware of chia and its many healthful components, so in order to make sure they do not make a mistake, they err on the safe side and tend not to recommend it. Unfortunate as this may be, it is an outgrowth of the current state of litigation in the U.S.

BACKGROUND & HISTORY

Q. What is chia?

A. Chia seed (*Salvia hispanica* L.) is a member of the mint family and originated in southern Mexico and Guatemala. Although people commonly refer to it as chia, what they are really referring to is the seed of the plant.

Q. Is chia a grain?

A. Though it can be used like a grain—including grinding it into a product similar to flour, which can be used in baking—chia is technically a seed. More specifically, it is an oilseed, since the seed contains more than 30 percent oil.

Q. Where does the name "chia" come from?

A. There are several versions of this story. The Aztec word for chia was "chian," which means "oily." When the word was translated from Nahuatl, the native language of the Aztecs, it was shortened. Interestingly, the present-day Mexican state of Chiapas comes from the Nahuatl place-name Chiapan, which comes from *chia* and *apan*, meaning "chia river" or "chia water."

The botanical name for chia, *Salvia hispanica*, was given by famed botanist Carl Linnaeus (1707–1778). Salvia is the genus name for the mint family, of which chia is a member. *Hispanica* is the Latin word for Spain. It is theorized that after the Spanish conquest of Mexico, the mysterious seeds were introduced to the Spanish countryside in about 1521, where they soon began to grow wild. Linnaeus mistakenly classified chia as a native Spanish species.

Q. How is chia related to the Aztecs?

A. Chia was the third most important crop for the Aztecs. They had four main crops: corn, beans, chia, and amaranth. The Aztecs knew about chia's many properties, and grew a number of different types of chia, each selected for its specific properties. They used chia as a food for themselves as well as their animals, and also used it for medicinal purposes and in religious ceremonies. These practices are documented in the codices written 500 years ago when the Spanish conquered the Aztecs.

Chia was virtually lost for five centuries after the Spanish conquest (due to both religious and agronomic reasons). This changed in the 1990s because of an effort lead by the University of Arizona to establish new crops in northwestern Argentina. This project led to the successful commercialization of chia as a crop, making it more widely available today.

Q. Where did Aztecs get chia?

A. Chia is native to the regions of Mexico and Central America inhabited by the Aztecs. However, according to Aztec mythology, chia seed arrived directly from the nose of Cinteotl, the maize god.

Q. Given the importance of chia to the Aztecs, why did it disappear?

A. The disappearance of chia seems to coincide with the arrival of Hernán Cortés and the conquistadors. The Aztecs, who ate chia and used it as medicine, believed it gave them mystical, almost supernatural, energy and power. Cortez felt that if he could destroy the crop, he could overpower the Aztecs and establish Spanish rule.

Further, based on the research I have done, chia was used in Aztec religious ceremonies as an offering to the gods—much like communion. In an attempt to replace the Aztec's religion with Christianity, the friars appeared to have outlawed chia. Lastly, the Spanish were interested in producing crops they were familiar with. Since chia couldn't grow in Europe, they considered it to be of no value. The only reason it survived is because a few people took the seed into the mountains where they continued to grow it for their own use.

Q. Did the Mayans eat chia?

A. Although chia grew wild and may have been used as a refreshing drink by the Mayans, it appears as if chia was only cultivated toward the end of Mayan civilization, around 800 A.D. This is when the Mayans began abandoning their cities and the Aztecs were consolidating their empire in central Mexico. So while the Mayans may (or may not) have consumed small amounts of chia, it was not an important food staple for them.

Q. How was chia rediscovered?

A. I was working on an agriculture project in northwestern Argentina aimed at identifying potential alternative crops for farmers. Chia was one of a number of seeds we planted in test plots. Because it grew so well, we started looking at how it might be used, its beneficial commercial properties, and also how to produce it commercially. From that research we went on to produce chia commercially, market it, and to educate the public on its wonderful health benefits.

Q. Where does chia come from?

A. Originally, chia was grown in the land of the Aztecs: central Mexico and Guatemala. Today, chia is grown commercially in most

Latin American countries, from Mexico to Argentina. There is even some chia production in Australia. Typically chia needs to be grown between 23 degrees north and south latitude.

Q. Are there different varieties of chia?
A. Technically there is only one variety of chia. Claims are made to the contrary, but these are just claims. In actuality there are different selections. For example if you pull the white seed out of common chia and plant it, you will get white seed. Plant the black seeds and you get black seeds. Oil and omega-3 content, protein, and phytonutrients vary somewhat between the colors, but not significantly.

Q. I've heard there are different colors of chia seed. What's the difference?
A. There are two chia seed colors, white and black. A popular brand of white chia is Salba, a white chia seed grown in Peru. The difference between the two colors, however, is negligible. I prefer the black seed because, just as darkly colored fruits and vegetables contain higher levels of antioxidants than their pale cousins, dark chia seed contains higher levels of antioxidants than white. But in truth, both colors contain essentially the same amount of omega-3, protein, fiber, and other nutrients.

Q. I recently bought chia and it had a lot of brown seeds. What are these?
A. Good question! Brown seeds are either weed seeds or immature chia seeds. The weed seeds can impart a strong flavor to chia. Brown chia seeds are low in omega-3 and protein content, indicating that the quality of the chia is poor. Avoid chia that has brown seeds.

Q. It seems there are three ways to use and consumer chia: ground, whole, or mixed with water to create a gel. Is one of these forms of chia best?
A. Whatever is going to help you consume chia daily—or at least on a regular basis—is best. In other words, it depends on your personal preferences, and how you are most likely to use chia. Gels are great to stir into drinks or creamy foods, such as oatmeal, pudding, or peanut butter. I personally love the seeds, because they add crunch to sandwiches and salads. Ground (or milled) chia is terrific for baking. (Using chia in baked

goods is also a great way to "hide" it from children who are averse to eating anything "healthy." They'll never know!) Any form of chia, whether it's eaten whole, milled, or as a gel, contains the same nutrients and benefits.

Q. What factors affect chia quality?

A. Harvesting is one key factor. Harvesting the crop before it is mature leads to lower total oil and omega-3 contents and this can affect other components as well, such as protein, fiber, and nutrients.

Q. Does climate and location affect composition?

A. As with any oilseed crop, cool climates increase oil content. In the case of chia, this also means that the omega-3 content increases. The amount of rainfall, time of rainfall, soil conditions, etc. will also affect composition.

Q. What kind of conditions are best for growing chia?

A. A hardy plant, chia likes relatively arid conditions and warm to hot temperatures. It thrives in open, grassy areas of woodlands, as in desert areas and in sandy soil.

Q. Do bees like chia flowers?

A. Yes, as do ants.

Q. Can I go into my kitchen, pull out my bag of chia, plant a few seeds, and grown my own chia?

A. You could. With the appropriate conditions (soil, water, and heat), the chia seeds will sprout.

Q. Can chia be grown in little pots outside, or under lights indoors?

A. Chia can be grown inside near a bright window or under grow lights, or outside in full sun. Growing the seed is easy; it will sprout in pots placed outside, or on a paper towel that is kept wet.

Q. Will chia in pots produce edible seeds in an average growing season?

A. Ah, now here is the challenge! Producing edible seeds requires not only appropriate conditions (soil, water, and heat), but also sufficient agronomic know how and experience. To get a plant to flower and produce seeds, the plant needs tropical or subtropical weather, sandy soil, and a relatively stable supply of water. Chia will flower only when the days are short, so if it is planted outside of tropical areas, frost will damage the flowers and prevent the formation or maturation of the seed. It's probably easier to buy already harvested chia!

Q. Can I plant the chia—that I eat every morning—in my chia pet planters?

A. Yes. You can, if you'd like. However, the age of the seed and the conditions under which it has been stored, can dramatically reduce the viability, hence the germination rate of the seed.

Q. Can I sprout chia?

A. Yes, you can—in the very same way that you sprout alfalfa, mung beans, and other sprouts. You can either use a sprouter or sprinkle a teaspoon of seeds on a damp paper towel, making sure to mist it occasionally so that the seeds don't dry out. It will take about three or four days.

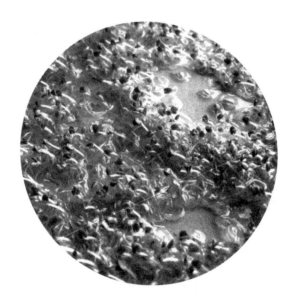

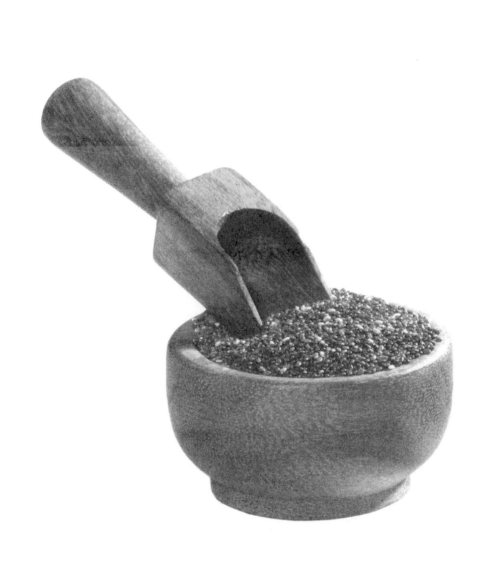

RESOURCES

BOOKS

COOKING WITH CHIA & OTHER FUNCTIONAL FOODS

The 100 Foods You Should Be Eating
by Glen Matten (New Holland, 2010)
This informative book hails from the UK, where it has been lauded for its practical, light-hearted approach to healthy eating. A fantastic choice for families.

The 100 Best Gluten-Free Recipes for Your Vegan Kitchen
by Kelly Keough (Ulysses Press, 2011).
A healthy look at getting the gluten and meat out of your kitchen. Chia is included!

Clean Food: A Seasonal Guide to Eating Close to the Source with More Than 200 Recipes for a Healthy and Sustainable You
by Terry Walters (Sterling Epicure, 2009).
More than a cookbook, this is a feast for the senses that will nourish mind, body, soul— and the planet, too.

The Complete Guide to Gluten-Free & Dairy-Free Cooking
by Glenis Lucas (Watkins, 2008).
With over 200 recipes, this informative cookbook features delicious, easy meals for improving health.

Cooking with Chia
by Gloria Hoover (Lulu.com, 2010).
Another non-health book (recipes include Bisquick-mix pancakes) that provides many fun ways to add chia to your meals.

The Food Doctor: Healing Foods for Mind and Body
by Vicki Edgson and Ian Marber (Collins & Brown, 2004).
Research, recipes, and information about eating for one's body type and lifestyle. Full of case studies, advice, and food cures.

Green for Life
by Victoria Boutenko (North Atlantic Books, 2010).
Raw food chef Victoria Boutenko offers loads of raw veggie recipes, plus quite a number of pages devoted to chia.

Green Market Baking Book: 100 Delicious Recipes for Naturally Sweet & Savory Treats
by Laura C. Martin (Sterling, 2011).
Lose the sugar with recipes that use only natural sweeteners and seasonal products. Celebrity chefs from across the U.S. contribute their favorite recipes, many of them gluten-free, vegan, or low-fat.

The Green Southwest Cookbook, Fresh, Zesty, Sustainable
by Janet E. Taylor (Rio Nuevo Publishers, 2012). This important cookbook features health-supportive recipes using traditional Southwestern ingredients.

Natural Wonderfoods
by Paula Bartimeus (Duncan Baird, 2011). As you'll learn in this colorful book, good nutrition can enhance our memory and moods, counter the effects of aging, and ease common illnesses. These 100 wonder foods are the key to optimum health.

Nourish: Delicious Goodness for Every Stage of Life
by Jane Clarke (Collins & Brown, 2011). Here's how to nourish yourself in each stage of life with simple, nutrient-dense recipes.

Pastrymaking and Baking with Chia
by Vilma Lo Presti (De Los Cuatrovientos, 2009). Not a diet book by any means, but a sweet look at all the ways you can add chia to your life.

The Power of Ancient Foods
by Gene Spiller and Rowena Hubbard (Book Publishing Company, 2003). A look at the traditional foods of ancient civilizations. Chia isn't a main player in this healthy recipe collection, but wins our vote for best supporting actor.

The 10 Secrets of 100% Healthy People Cookbook
by Patrick Holford (Piatkus, 2009). A cookbook incorporating the diet secrets of the super healthy, with lots of recipes giving innovative ways of using chia seeds in both savory and sweet dishes.

Thrive Foods: 200 Plant-Based Recipes for Peak Health
by Brendan Brazier (Da Capo Lifelong Books, 2011). Another healthy recipe book that mentions chia.

The Top 100 Fitness Foods: 100 Ways to Turbocharge Your Life
by Sarah Owen (Duncan Baird, 2010). The first step to getting in shape is taking responsibility for your health—and the nutritionally balanced information in this book will help you do just that.

The Top 100 Healing Foods: 100 Foods to Relieve Common Ailments and Enhance Health and Vitality
by Paula Bartimeus (Duncan Baird, 2009). If you suffer from an ailment, are plagued by stress or insomnia, or are tired all the time, these natural wonder foods can help!

Welcoming Kitchen: 200 Delicious Allergen- & Gluten-Free Vegan Recipes
by Kim Lutz with Megan Hart (Sterling, 2011). Eat safe and delicious with these gluten and allergy-free vegan recipes.

Wild About Greens: 125 Delicious Recipes from Hearty Soups & Stews to Succulent Sautés and Smoothies
by Nava Atlas (Sterling, 2012)
It is easier than ever to incorporate the most nutritious foods on earth into delicious everyday fare.

SUPERFOODS, WHOLE FOODS & CHIA

Chia Cheat Sheet Chart
by Angela Stokes (The Raw Food World).
More a chart than a book, this book provides "at a glance" benefits and tips for using chia.

The Encyclopedia of Healing Foods
by Michael Murray and Joseph Pizzorno (Atria Press, 2005).
A close look at the power of foods to make you feel better, as well as heal specific ailments.

The Essential Herbs Handbook: More than 100 Herbs for Well-Being, Healing and Happiness
by Lesley Bremness
(Duncan Baird, 2009).
Over 100 life-enriching herbs are catalogued, with comprehensive references and information about each, including its Latin name, traditional uses, optimal growing conditions, and benefits to the body and mind.

Everything Superfoods Book: Discover What to Eat to Look Younger, Live Longer and Enjoy Life to the Fullest
by Delia Quigley (Adams Media, 2009).
This book breaks down the secrets of the top 20 superfoods and how they can be instrumental in transforming the body.

Healing Foods for Dummies
by Molly Siple (For Dummies, 1999).
An accessible introduction to the world of healing foods medicine. This is a fun, fact-filled resource for anyone looking for a safe, easy-to-use alternative or supplement to conventional medicine—and who looks forward to a long, healthy life.

Healing Plants Bible: The Definitive Guide to Herbs, Trees and Flowers
by Helen Farmer-Knowles (Sterling, 2010).
Plants used in organic medicine across the centuries and around the world, including Western herbalism, traditional Chinese medicine, and India's Ayurveda.

Healing With Whole Foods: Asian Traditions and Modern Nutrition
by Paul Pitchford
(North Atlantic Books, 2003).
This encyclopedic volume is a time-honored resource among naturopaths, holistic nutritionists, acupuncturists, and other holistic types. Some recipes.

Healing Spices: How to Use 50 Everyday and Exotic Spices to Boost Health and Beat Disease
by Bharat B. Aggarwal, with Deborah Yost (Sterling, 2011).
Studies of dietary patterns around the world confirm that spice-consuming populations have the lowest incidence of such life-threatening illnesses as heart disease, cancer, diabetes, and Alzheimer's.

Healthified Cooking: A Health and Wellness Book
by Caroline Driscoll (Fastpirnt Plus).
Easy to prepare recipes that support a healthy lifestyle. Well worth owning. It can be found at **http://www.healthifiedcooking.com**

How Can I Use Herbs in My Daily Life?
by Isabell Shipard
(David Stewart Books, 2003).
Easy ways to use nutritious, healing herbs in your current diet.

The New Complete Guide to Nutritional Health: More than 600 Foods and Recipes for Overcoming Illness & Boosting Your Immunity
by Pierre Cousin and Kirsten Hartvig (Duncan Baird, 2011).
From medicinal herbs to superfoods that reduce stress, ease pain, and boost the immune system, all the basic principles of good nutrition are outlined here.

Nutrition for Dummies
by Carol Ann Rinzler (For Dummies, 2011).
Discusses vitamins, minerals, fat content, carbohydrates, and more, prescribing practical ways to incorporate more nutritious eating into everyday life.

The New Whole Foods Encyclopedia: A Comprehensive Resource for Healthy Eating
by Rebecca Wood (Penguin, 2010).
Provides an alphabetical listing of more than 1,000 whole foods: grains, vegetables, fruits, nuts, seeds, seaweeds, fungi, sweeteners, fats, oils, herbs, and spices. Entries include historical information, health benefits, uses, and buying guidelines.

Superfoods HealthStyle: Proven Strategies for Lifelong Health
by Steven Pratt, M.D. and Kathy Matthews (Harper Paperback, 2006).
Your guide to a longer, healthier, better life, it translates the most recent cutting-edge research into simple recommendations that you can use to vastly improve your physical and mental health.

Super Immunity Foods
by Frances Sheridan Goulart (McGraw Hill, 2009).
Incorporate foods into your diet that build immunity, beat disease, and slow aging.

The Whole-Food Guide to Overcoming Irritable Bowel Syndrome: Strategies and Recipes for Eating Well with IBS, Indigestion and Other Digestive Disorders
by Laura Knoff
(New Harbinger Publications, 2010).
This fantastic book includes chia as a way to soothe chronic digestive issues.

RUNNING, FITNESS & CHIA

90-Day Fitness Journal
by Rose Sery (Sterling Innovation, 2010).
A 90-day journal that helps users track their workouts, their eating plan, and their speedy progress.

Anatomy for Strength and Fitness Training: An Illustrated Guide to Your Muscles in Action
by Mark Vella (McGraw Hill, 2006).
A magnificent visual insight into what happens to your muscles when you exercise. By understanding how your body responds to each movement, you'll be able to isolate specific muscle groups and design the most targeted program possible.

The Beginning Runner's Handbook: The Proven 13-Week Run-Walk Program
by Ian MacNeill (Greystone Books, 2005).
The injury-free way to take up running.

Born to Run
by Christopher McDougall
(Vintage Press, 2011).
Journalist Christopher McDougall visits a mysterious people in the Chiapas area of Mexico who share their secrets for ultra-distance races. (Chia is one of their go-to foods.)

The Complete Book of Sports Nutrition: A Practical Guide to Eating for Sport
by Shelly Meltzer and Cecily Fuller
(New Holland, 2007).
Every sport has its own metabolic needs and its own dietary requirements, as the authors of this practical, scientifically sound book explain. Starting with the basics of a balanced diet, they recommend combinations of foods and eating plans that deliver the ideal proportions of proteins, carbohydrates, fats, vitamins, and minerals for each type of sport.

The Everything Running Book: The Ultimate Guide to Injury-Free Running for Fitness and Competition
by Art Liberman, Randy Brown, and Eileen Myers (Adams Media, 2012).
Cutting-edge information on hugely influential trends in natural running, selecting the right gear, managing your nutrition, and the diets favored by endurance athletes.

The Life You Want: Get Motivated,
Lose Weight, and Be Happy
by Bob Greene, Ann Kearney-Cooke PhD,
and Janis Jibrin RD (Simon & Schuster, 2010).
Fitness, diet, and psychological support, all
in one book.

The Men's Health Big Book of Exercise:
Four Weeks to a Leaner, Stronger,
More Muscular You
by Adam Campbell, (Rodale Books, 2009).
This 480-page muscle manual bulges with
hundreds of useful tips, the latest findings in
exercise science, and cutting-edge workouts
from the world's top trainers.

The Power of Your Prime: A Doctor's Secrets to
Men's Health and Peak Performance for Life
by Florence Comite, (Rodale Books, 2012).
As a man ages, a slow decline takes root im-
perceptibly and day-by-day: fat around the
middle, low energy, dull mental skills, less-
ened libido. Here, readers learn how to get
back what they've lost, restore vitality and
health, prevent (and even reverse) disease,
and feel better than ever before.

Push: 30 Days to Turbocharged Habits,
a Bangin' Body and the Life You Deserve!
by Chalene Johnson (Rodale Books, 2011).
How to supersize your motivation and create
an accountability system to achieve any fitness (or life) goal you desire.

Super Body, Super Brain
by Michael Gonzalez-Wallace
(HarperOne, 2010).
How to harness the brain's support to get fit.

Which Comes First, Cardio or Weights?
Fitness Myths, Training Truths, and Other
Surprising Discoveries from the Science of
Exercise
by Alex Hutchinson
(Harper Paperback, 2011).
This myth-busting book covers the full spec-
trum of exercise science and offers the latest
in research from around the globe, as well as
helpful diagrams and plenty of practical tips
on using proven science to improve fitness,
reach weight loss goals, and achieve better
competition results.

GENERAL HEALTH

50 Ways to Soothe Yourself Without Food
by Susan Albers
(New Harbinger Publications, 2009).
Lose your dependence on eating as a means
of coping with difficult emotions.

Clean Body: The Humble Art of Zen-
Cleansing Yourself
by Michael DeJong (Sterling, 2009).
Embodies a mindset, a philosophy—an alternative to mass consumerism. DeJong draws
from Eastern belief systems—especially the
element theory in Chinese medicine and

Asian cooking—and harmoniously balances five pure essentials in his recipes, using baking soda, lemon, olive oil, salt, and white vinegar as the basis for his all-natural concoctions.

Clean Cures: The Humble Art of Zen-Curing Yourself
by Michael DeJong (Sterling, 2009).
Why use strong chemicals to treat minor ailments when there are safe, natural, and effective remedies that relieve everything from aching muscles to toothaches to acne?

The End of Overeating: Taking Control of the Insatiable American Appetite
by David Kessler (Rodale, 2010).
A former FDA commissioner describes how, since the 1980s, the food industry, acting with the advertising industry and lifestyle changes, have left many individuals addicted to eating.

Encyclopedia of Natural Medicine
by Michael Murray and Joseph Pizzorno, (Three Rivers Press, 1997).
An in-depth look at the power of alternative healing therapies to help keep you healthy.

The Feel Good Factor
by Patrick Holford, Piatkus (Piatkus, 2010).
A book on how to improve your mood and motivation, reduce anxiety and get a good night's sleep.

Folks, This Ain't Normal
by Joel Salatin
(Center Street, 2011).
A discussion of how far removed we are from the land, and how that has affected modern-day health.

Food Matters: A Guide to Conscious Eating with More Than 75 Recipes
by Mark Bittman
(Simon & Schuster, 2009).
Explains how the food we eat is doing damage to our bodies and the environment, and the changes we need to make.

Food Rules: An Eater's Manual
by Michael Pollan and Maira Kalman
(Penguin, 2011).
Short, sweet, and easy to read, this may be one of the best "how to eat healthy" manuals on the market. A classic.

Live Better, Live Longer: The New Studies That Reveal What's Really Good—and Bad—For Your Health
by Sanjiv Chopra and Alan Lotvin
(St. Martin's Griffin, 2010).
A look at the research on health and aging.

Natural Health, Natural Medicine
by Andrew Weil (Mariner Books, 2004).
A holistic health favorite from the good doctor Weil.

Nuts and Seeds in Health and Disease Prevention (Chapter 38)
by Wayne Coates
(Academic Press, 2011).
An in-depth look at the healing power of chia and other seeds.

The 10 Secrets of Healthy Aging
by Patrick Holford & Jerome Burne
(Piatkus, 2012).
Explores how to age well and stay healthy throughout your life. It talks about the importance of superfoods, including chia.

Wild-Type Food in Health Promotion and Disease Prevention (Chapter 26)
by Ricardo Ayerza and Wayne Coates
(Humana Press, 2010).
Explores the importance of biodiversity and alternative plant foods in the prevention of disease.

What to Eat
by Marion Nestle (North Point Press, 2007).
Consume fewer calories, exercise more, eat more fruits and vegetables, and eliminate junk food. The key to eating well, Nestle advises, is to learn to navigate through the aisles in large supermarkets. To that end, she gives readers a virtual tour, highlighting the main concerns of each food group, including baby food, health foods, and prepared foods and supplements.

Why We Get Fat: And What to Do About It
by Gary Taubes (Knopf, 2011).
A science journalist explains why Americans are so fat.

Worried Sick: A Prescription for Health in an Overtreated America
by Nortin M. Hadler
(University of North Carolina Press, 2008).
Learn to take control of your own health by distinguishing between sound medical advice and persuasive medical marketing.

You: The Owner's Manual
by Michael Roizen and Mehmet Oz
(William Morrow, 2008).
We still love this classic for simplifying how the body works—and how to best take care of it.

HISTORY

The Aztec Calendar Handbook
by Randall C. Jiminez and Richard B. Graeber
(Historical Science Publishing, 2001).
Myths, gods, and day-to-day life of this fascinating culture.

Aztec Thought and Culture: A Study of the Ancient Nahuatl Mind
by Miguel Leion-Portilla
(University of Oklahoma Press, 1990).
A look at the Nahuatl codices and folios of the Aztecs.

The Aztecs: Peoples of America
by Michael E. Smith
(Wiley Blackwell, 2002).
A thorough examination of Aztec origins and civilization that covers religion, science, and thought.

Chia: Rediscovering a Forgotten Crop of the Aztecs
by Ricardo Ayerza and Wayne Coates
(The University of Arizona Press, 2005).

Daily Life of the Aztecs
by David Carrasco and Scott Sessions
(Greenwood Press, 2011).
A look at the traditions and everyday ways of the great Aztecs.

Fifteen Poets of the Aztec World
by Miguel Leon-Portilla
(University of Oklahoma Press, 2000).
The exquisite poetic tradition of Nahuatl speakers of the central Mexican highlands.

History and Mythology of the Aztecs: The Codex Chimalpopoca
by John Bierhorst
(University of Arizona Press, 1998).
The rise of the Aztecs, including their myths and pre-Cortesian history.

Mexico: The Signs of History
by Pietro Tarallo
(White Star Publishers, 2010).

From the Olmecs to the Toltecs, from the Mayans to the Aztecs, to the conquistadores who liberated Mexico from Spain, Mexico is a crossroads of cultures and artistic expressions.

Victors and Vanquished: Spanish and Nahua Views of the Conquest of Mexico
by Stuart B. Schwartz (St. Martin's, 2000).
Learn how personal interests, class and ethnic biases, and political considerations influenced the history of Mexico.

INTERNET
COOKING WITH CHIA & OTHER FUNCTIONAL FOODS

http://www.101cookbooks.com
A terrific recipe website using whole food ingredients, including chia.

http://www.azchia.com
This is Dr. Wayne Coates's own website, chock-full of the latest research, discoveries, studies, recipes, and chia lore. A must-see resource for anyone who cares about his or her health.

http://www.beyondsalmon.com
Cooking instructions and recipes for salmon, quinoa, and plenty of veggies.

http://www.cookingchia.com/en
This is Vilma Lo Presti's website, where her book, *Pastrymaking and Baking with Chia*, is featured. Plenty of information on chia.

http://www.cookingquinoa.net/
The place to go to learn how to make quinoa—as well as make a number of great dishes containing quinoa.

http://glutenfreegoddess.blogspot.com/
High-nutrient, gluten-free recipes featuring quinoa, chia, and other power-packed ingredients.

http://www.healthygreenkitchen.com/
Amaranth, coconut oil, chia, quinoa—we love this blog!

http://www.localharvest.org/
Looking for a local farmer? Farmer's market? CSA (Community Supported Agriculture)? Or simply want to know what's in season in your area? Go to LocalHarvest to find out.

http://ohsheglows.com/
Another great website with superfood recipes, including chia.

http://www.quinoatips.com/
Another terrific quinoa cooking website!

http://www.rawfoodrecipes.com/recipes/category/chia.html
This raw cooking website has many interesting looking (and healthy) chia recipes. The Orange Chia Seed Breakfast Pudding is great!

http://www.savvyvegetarian.com/
Great, nutrient-dense recipes, many packed with superfoods.

http://www.wholefoodsmarket.com/recipes/
Whole Foods Market's website is loaded with excellent recipes—including some with chia!

SUPERFOODS, WHOLE FOODS & CHIA

http://allfoodsnatural.com/
This pretty website has recipes, natural foods resources, and recipes—as well as a cooking club to help you upgrade your whole-food cooking quotient.

http://www.naturalnews.com/
NaturalNews is packed with articles, tips, references, videos, podcasts, cartoons, and even music—all in the name of good health.

http://www.fruitsandveggiesmatter.gov/
Run by the Centers for Disease Control, this fun and interactive website makes it easy to learn how to get the vegetables and fruits your body needs.

http://greenforlife.com/
Raw food, green food, vegetable smoothies, and more.

http://greensmoothiesblog.com/
Green smoothies are one of the easiest ways to get your veggies. This website is dedicated to the nutrient-dense drink.

http://www.montereybayaquarium.org/cr/seafoodwatch.aspx
Monterey Bay Aquarium's famous "Seafood Watch" helps consumers choose safe, low-metal seafood that is not endangered. Good for your body, good for the planet.

http://www.nutritionalresearch.org/
Packed with links to nutrition research studies as well as other resources. A must-visit website!

http://www.StephaniePedersen.com
Co-author Stephanie Pedersen's home website.

http://www.superfoodsrx.com
This commercial website has a plethora of information on favorite high impact foods, as well as nutrients, a collection of research, and an up-to-the-minute blog.

http://userealbutter.com/
This gorgeous, tasty website espouses eating real foods, including superfoods such as kale and quinoa. Fantastic recipes.

http://www.whfoods.com
Billing itself as "the world's healthiest foods," WHFoods.com is an awesome collection of whole, super, and functional foods, with plenty of research studies, nutrient profiles, allergy info, habitat and history, and cultural background for each food. Highly recommended.

RUNNING, FITNESS & CHIA

http://www.fasttracktofatloss.com/
Free online fitness training and accountability coaching.

http://www.fitness.com/
A comprehensive library of workouts, advice, education, and recipes.

http://www.fitwoman.com/blog/
Join in and learn what you can do to help get fit.

http://healthresearch.lbl.gov/
The National Runners' Health Study began in 1991. Check in to see what research is currently being conducted, and what has been learned about running and fitness.

http://www.itrain.com/
Downloadable workouts from celebrity trainers. Load your iPod and get moving.

http://www.lovingfit.com/
Food, supplements, and routines for a more fit you.

http://www.myoptumhealth.com
Optimizing health and well-being, this website is a fitness fiend's dream. A generous smattering of food, alternative therapy, and medical information is an added draw.

http://www.nutrition.gov
This is the U.S. government's fitness and health website. Lots of resources on lots of health and fitness topics.

http://runningtimes.com/
Running Times is America's most popular running magazine. Take a look and see why. Health articles, race listings, product reviews, training strategies, and more.

http://running.about.com/
About.com's running and jogging website is a massive collection of articles. No matter how seasoned you are, what type of running you do, or on what terrain, there is something here for you. This website can send you to many other places.

http://www.runnersworld.com/shoeadvisor
Find the perfect pair of athletic shoes—just enter your vitals.

http://www.trainwithmeonline.com/
A mostly free website featuring exercise routines, fitness help, customized workouts, and online training groups.

GENERAL HEALTH

http://www.diet-blog.com
Diet news and research, rolled into one handy blog.

http://www.doctoroz.com/
Dr. Mehmet Oz's website.

http://www.eatwellguide.org
Finding local, seasonal food just got easier. Plug in your zip code and—voila! Farms, markets, restaurants, and more throughout the U.S. and Canada.

http://www.edf.org/
The Environmental Defense Fund helps individuals avoid environmental pollution in the air, food supply, and everywhere else.

http://www.ewg.org/foodnews/
The Environmental Working Group is famous for its regularly updated "dirty dozen" and "clean fifteen" lists, which help shoppers decide where they can save by purchasing safe mainstream produce, and where it is essential to go organic.

http://www.fitness.gov
This is the official website for The President's Council on Fitness, Sports & Nutrition.

http://www.foodandwaterwatch.org/blogs/
A look into the politics and players of today's food industries.

http://www.healthfinder.gov
The U.S. Government's health website, featuring links, resources, and education.

http://www.mayoclinic.com
The famous Mayo Clinic's health education website.

http://www.mealsmatter.org
The tagline of Meals Matter is Meal Planning Made Simple. Aimed at busy families and using plenty of familiar (often mainstream) ingredients, this fun website is a great resource for those just easing into a healthier lifestyle.

http://www.medicinenet.com
An easy-to-use source of information on a wide range of conditions, including symptom checkers, and nutritional support.

http://www.rodaleinstitute.org
We love Rodale's focus on chemical-free farming, their strong stand against global warming, and the generous nutrition information.

http://www.naturalnews.com/
NaturalNews is packed with articles, tips, references, videos, podcasts, cartoons, and even music—all in the name of good health.

http://www.webmd.com
The online source of health and slightly holistic medical advice.

HISTORY

http://www.azchia.com/chia_seed_history.htm
AZChia is Dr. Wayne Coates's website, where you can learn about how the Incas and others lifted chia from a food staple to a sacred gift to the gods.

http://www.aztec-history.com
This website has an exhaustive amount of information on the Aztecs.

http://www.aztec-indians.com/
A simple website with a wide range of information on Aztecs.

http://aztecs.mrdonn.org
Plenty of history and cultural information on the Aztecs and pre-Spanish Mexico. A terrific website for kids.

http://www.foodtimeline.org/foodmaya.html
An intensive timeline that includes common Aztec meals, dining customs, and even a chocolate recipe.

http://www.history-aztec.com
Another well-researched website on Aztec culture and history.

http://casademexico.com/
The history of Mexico, including early peoples and pre-Spanish history.

http://worldhistory.pppst.com/aztecs.html
A great website about the Aztecs for kids.

RESEARCH AND STUDIES

http://www.azchia.com/research
Over the last couple decades, chia has been heavily researched—and the studies continue. Here, you'll find links to all of the essential technical studies on chia that have been done.

PUBLICATIONS

http://www.cleaneatingmag.com
Clean Eating is a newcomer to the world of magazines. It is aimed at taking you beyond the food you eat to explore the multitude of health and nutritional benefits of living a clean lifestyle.

http://www.cookinglight.com
A favorite of calorie counters and long-term dieters, *Cooking Light* makes your favorite foods less caloric.

http://www.eatingwell.com
One of our favorite magazines, *Eating Well* talks health from the plate up. Filled with whole foods recipes, health articles, research, and personal essays.

http://www.fitnessmagazine.com
Fitness magazine has all kinds of exercise and get-fit advice, with a healthy dose of diet and nutrition information.

http://www.health.com
General health magazine with a fitness and diet focus.

http://www.livingwithout.com
Living Without is the go-to resource for anyone living with food allergies, sensitivities, or intolerances. Filled with cutting-edge research, as well as in-depth looks at specific food issues, it also features loads of wheat-free, dairy-free, and soy-free recipes, many of them containing chia.

http://www.mensfitness.com
With a strong emphasis on sculpting the body through weight lifting and exercise, *Men's Fitness* also has diet and nutrition advice.

http://www.menshealth.com
Published by Rodale Press, *Men's Health* is a mainstream fitness-oriented magazine with plenty of nutrition and weight loss advice.

http://www.naturalhealthmag.com
What began as a "hardcore" macrobiotic and spirituality publication has recently gone mainstream with advice on everything from mindset to healthy eating to green living.

http://www.prevention.com
Another Rodale Press publication, *Prevention* is the time-honored source of research-based diet, exercise, lifestyle, and nutrition information.

http://www.womenshealthmag.com
Published by Rodale Press, *Women's Health*, is a mainstream fitness-oriented magazine with plenty of nutrition and weight loss advice.

http://www.shape.com
Shape began as a fitness and diet magazine, heavy on aerobics. Today, it's grown to a healthy lifestyle publication aimed at helping women lose pounds and maintain their weight loss. Chia makes regular appearances in the recipe pages.

http://www.vegetariantimes.com
The *Vegetarian Times'* tagline is "Great Food, Good Health, Smart Living," which pretty much wraps up what this fun, informative magazine is all about. Both chia and Dr. Wayne Coates have been featured in the magazine.

http://www.vegnews.com
This magazines is aimed at hardcore vegans—but its health articles and recipes are great for everyone.

http://www.wholeliving.com
Created by the publishers of Martha Stewart Living, this magazine has an organic, holistic, green bent, which colors everything from its recipes to its fashion sections.

ORGANIZATIONS

http://www.eatright.org/
The American Dietetic Association is not the most progressive food education organization around, but they do provide solid information on calories, food groups, and basic nutrition.

http://www.eco-farm.org/
Nurturing healthy farms, food systems, and communities.

http://www.farmtoschool.org
Farm to School connects schools (K–12) and local farms with the objectives of serving healthy meals in school cafeterias; improving student nutrition; providing agriculture, health and nutrition education opportunities; and supporting local and regional farmers.

http://www.nourishingtheplanet.org
WorldWatch Institute's Nourish The Planet program is a nonprofit focused on highlighting environmentally sustainable ways of alleviating hunger and poverty.

http://www.nutrition.org/
The American Society for Nutrition stands for excellence in nutrition research and science.

http://www.organicconsumers.org/
The Organic Consumers Association helps maintain organic food standards.

http://www.panna.org/
The Pesticide Action Network provides information about harmful pesticides and works to replace pesticide use with ecologically sound and socially just alternatives.

http://www.slowfood.com/
Slow Food works to persevere traditional, cultural foods, recipes, and ways of eating.

http://www.sustainabletable.org
Sustainable Table celebrates local sustainable food and growing methods, as well as educates consumers on food-related issues.

http://truefoodnow.org/
The True Food Network's Center for Food Safety works to protect human health and the environment by curbing the proliferation of harmful food production technologies and by promoting organic and other forms of sustainable agriculture.

METRIC CONVERSION CHART

VOLUME

1 teaspoon	5 ml
1 tablespoon	15 ml
¼ cup	60 ml
⅓ cup	80 ml
⅔ cup	160 ml
¾ cups	180 ml
1 cup	240 ml
1 pint	475 ml
1 quart	.95 liter
1 quart plus ¼ cup	1 liter
1 gallon	3.8 liters

TEMPERATURE

32°F	0°C
212°F	100°C
250°F	121°C
325°F	163°C
350°F	176°C
375°F	190°C
400°F	205°C
425°F	218°C
450°F	232°C

To convert from Fahrenheit to Celsius:
Subtract 32, multiply by 5, then divide by 9.

WEIGHT

1 ounce	28.3 grams
4 ounces	113 grams
8 ounces	227 grams
12 ounces	340.2 grams

Excerpted from *The Good Housekeeping Cookbook* (Hearst Books/Sterling Publishing).

ACKNOWLEDGMENTS

Ricardo Ayerza, who lives in Buenos Aires, Argentina, has been a friend and collaborator for 30 years. We have worked together for many years studying many new crops, including chia, while traveling extensively in South America. His friendship and knowledge helped to greatly advance our research with chia and the other new crops we worked on.

Patricia Coates (1950–2004), my wife of 34 years, passed away suddenly in 2004. Her support throughout my career at The University of Arizona, while researching new crops, and especially chia, was instrumental in keeping me going during my many absences from home. Her contribution is still missed.

Patricia Wiercinski, whom I married in 2006, has been extremely supportive of my work with chia, and is a valued partner in our business, AZChia. Her help with the everyday operation of the company, as well as her support through many trying times, is greatly appreciated. I would not be where I am today without her continued support and encouragement.

Additionally, I would like to thank the many people who have interacted with me during the 20 years I have been researching, commercializing, and bringing chia to the marketplace. This includes farmers, growers, university researchers, and business entities. Their support and encouragement has helped bring chia to the the status it enjoys today in terms of helping improve the health of many individuals.

We would like to thank Marcus Leaver and Michael Fragnito for helping share the word about chia. Their enthusiasm for chia is what brought this book into existence. We are very appreciative of their support—which has made it possible for more people to learn about this important superfood.

INDEX

Note: Page numbers *in italics* indicate recipes.

A

Acid tamer, 85

Alcohol, 25–26, 70, 133, 135

Allergies, chia and, 20, 156

Aloe, squeezing, 119. *See also* Beauty recipes

Alpha-linolenic acid (ALA), 7, 11, 15, 28, 135–136, 146, 147, 152, 156

Amaranth, 44, 97

Amino acids, 12–13, 17, 44, 78, 99, 148, 149, 153. *See also* Protein

Antioxidants. *See also* Omega-3 fatty acids
  avocados providing, 100
  in chia, 132
  chia providing, 7, 8, 32, 36, 38, 50, 124, 129, 145, 147–148, 150, 151, 160
  defined, 38
  oxidation and, 38, 152, 155
  storing chia and, 69, 154, 155
  strengthening immune system, 142
  vitamins and minerals, 18, 19

Arthritis, 42, 148

Avocados
  about: nutritional value and benefits, 100
  Chia Guacamole, *101*
  Moisturizing Chia-Avocado Mask, *119*

Aztecs
  amaranth and, 44, 97
  chia history and, 8–9, 158–159
  chia name origin and, 158
  chia uses, 8–9, 14, 19, 20, 50, 58, 95, 141
  cultivating chia, 14, 68

B

Baked treats, 71–77
  about: baking times, 77; cake mixes, 75. *See also* Desserts; coating baked goods with chia seeds, 102; heating

chia and, 71; low-fat baking, 76; milled chia and, 71; without gluten, 74
  Banana Bread, *74*
  Chia Cornbread, *73*
  Chia Seed Muffins, *71*
  Chia Snack Bars, *76*
  Gluten-Free Chia Muffins, *72*
  Protein Muffins, *72–73*
  Pumpkin Bread, *75*

Banana Bread, *74*

Beans and legumes
  about: black beans, 107; fiber from, 107
  Chia Chipotle Bean Burger, *107*
  Chia Hummus, *90*
  Chia Meatloaf, *102*
  Chia Polenta with White Beans, *105–106*
  Chia Vegetarian Chili, *103*
  Lima Bean Winter Soup, *86*
  Mulligatawny Chia Soup, *88*

Beauty recipes, 119–122
  about: adding chia to beauty routine, 119; Aztecs and chia, 20; chia oil and, 150; Epsom salts and, 122; jojoba oil and, 121; nail care and, 122, 149–150; rose water and, 121; seaweed and, 120; skin health and, 8, 144–145; squeezing aloe for, 119
  Almond Face Scrub, *121*
  Chia Nail Treatment, *122*
  High Glow Scrub, *122*
  Kelp Face Pack, *120*
  Moisturizing Chia-Avocado Mask, *119*
  Skin Refreshing Mask, *120*
  Super Fast Face Pack I and II, *120–121*

Benefits of chia, 11–20
  about: overview of, 9
  brain, nervous system health and, 144
  cancer and. *See* Cancer

cardiovascular conditions and, 131–134. *See also* Cholesterol

diabetes and, 137–139, 149

digestive health and, 139–140, 148–149, 156

exercise and. *See* Exercise, endurance, and energy

fatigue and, 141

immune system and, 142–143

inflammation and. *See* Inflammation

Omega-3 fatty acid benefits, 7, 11, 15, 19, 27, 42, 129, 136, 141, 144

skin health and, 144–145. *See also* Beauty recipes

Berries

about: strawberries, 112

Berry Cloud Pudding, *111–112*

Beverages

about: drinking immediately, 68

Almond Delight, *66*

Basic Chia Protein Shake, *67*

Chia Fresca, *65*, 154

Citrus Julius, *67*

Fruit Slushy, *69*

Ginger Pear Eggnog Smoothie, *68*

Green Super Smoothie, *66*

Spicy Green Chocolate Shake, *69*

Tropical Champagne Punch Smoothie, *70*

Blood pressure

chia and, 29, 33, 36, 45, 131, 134, 156, 157

exercise and, 62, 133

heart disease and, 133, 134

Blood sugar levels

balancing/stabilizing, 18, 19, 24, 33, 112, 138, 149

raising, things to avoid, 25, 26

Body mass index (BMI), 23, 24

Brain and nervous system health, 144

Breads. *See* Baked treats

Breakfast, 77–85

about: chia egg toppers, 80; chia intake amounts, 28, 29, 41; fast chia breakfasts, 82; weight-loss menus by phase, 30–39; weight-maintenance menus, 41–45

Aussie-Style Broiled Tomatoes with Chia, *84–85*

Chia Breakfast Polenta, *106*

Chia Breakfast Syrup, *79*

Chia Frittata, *80*

Chia Gel, *77*

Chianola, *83–84*

Chia-Nut Butter Sandwich, *81*

Chia-Oat Porridge, *82*

Chia-Quinoa Porridge, *83*

Cinnamon-Orange Pancakes, *78*

French Chia Toast, *79*

Orange Date Syrup, *78–79*

Raw Vanilla Coconut "Yogurt," *81*

Scrambled Chia Eggs, *80*

Buckwheat, 44

Bunny drink, *124*

Burgers, *107–108*

C

Caffeine, 26

Calcium, 12, 18, 84, 97, 149–150

Canary Crunch, *123*

Cancer, 129–131

catching early, 142

colorectal, 56, 140, 147

exercise and, 56

facts, 130

lowering risk of, 7, 15, 19, 20, 100, 107, 112, 129

mechanics of, 129

phytonutrients and, 20, 129

prostate, chia and, 157

survivor testimonial, 131

Cardiovascular conditions, 131–134. *See also* Blood pressure; Cholesterol

Carrots

about: lore and trivia, 93, 118

Moist Carrot Cake, *117–118*

Moroccan Carrot Salad, *93*

Cat food, *124*

Cereals. *See* Breakfast

Cheese, in Chia Quesadillas, *100–101*

ABOUT THE AUTHORS

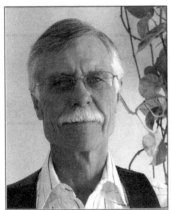

PATRICIA WIERCINSKI

DR. WAYNE COATES

Wayne Coates, PhD, is an ultra-distance runner who regularly runs races of up to 100 miles, helped along by daily doses of endurance-enhancing chia. An agricultural engineer, Dr. Coates is Professor Emeritus in the Office of Arid Lands Studies at The University of Arizona. He is the author of more than 60 articles in technical and agricultural journals. His work with chia began in 1990, when he traveled to Argentina to study the commercial potential for new crops. It was during this time that he developed the system currently used to harvest and clean chia seed. Founder of the educational chia website www.azchia.com, and head of AZChia's retail operation, Coates's current research activities are focused on making this health seed widely known and used throughout the world.

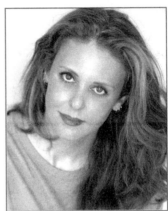

EDDIE MALLUK

STEPHANIE PEDERSEN

Stephanie Pedersen, CHHC, AADP, is a health writer and certified holistic health counselor. She works with busy entrepreneurs, professionals, and entertainment professionals to help them lose weight and improve their health so they can serve as many people as possible through their work. Pedersen currently lives in New York City with her husband and three sons. Visit Stephanie at **www.StephaniePedersen.com**.

PHOTOGRAPHY CREDITS